Compact Tai Chi

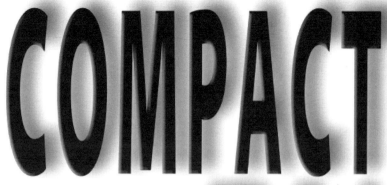

COMPACT TAI CHI

Combined forms for practice in limited space

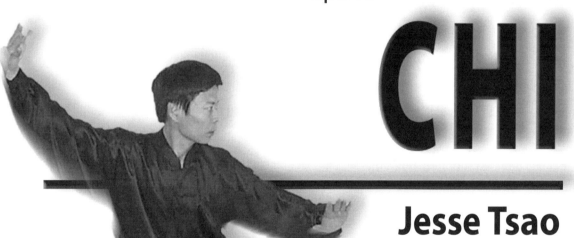

Jesse Tsao

Samuel Weiser, Inc.
York Beach, Maine

First published in 2000 by
Samuel Weiser, Inc.
Box 612
York Beach, Maine 03910-0612
www.weiserbooks.com

Library of Congress Cataloging-in-Publication Data

Tsao, Jesse
    Compact tai chi : combined forms to practice in a limited
space / Jesse Tsao.
      p. cm.
    ISBN 1-57863-126-2 (pbk. : alk. paper)
    1. T'ai chi ch'üan
    GV504.T83 2000
    613.7'148—dc21
                           99–058152

VG
Typeset in 9/12 Formata
Cover and interior photographs by Julia Z. Tsao
Cover and text design by Kathryn Sky-Peck

PRINTED IN THE UNITED STATES OF AMERICA

07 06 05 04 03 02 01 00
8 7 6 5 4 3 2 1

Contents

Introduction

Fundamental Techniques

Sequence 1

Sequence 2

Sequence 3

Sequence 4

发扬太极拳，
造福人民大众。

贺

凤山同学拳作出版

李德印

99年之月

Carry forward the Tai
Chi Tradition to Promote
the Well-Being of Mankind

—Professor Deyin Li

VICE CHAIRMAN OF BEIJING
WUSHU ASSOCIATION

TAI CHI DRILLMASTER OF THE
CHINESE NATIONAL WUSHU TEAM

FORMER CHIEF JUDGE OF THE
CHINESE NATIONAL
TAI CHI COMPETITION

Foreword

I vividly recall the first time seeing and experiencing Jesse Tsao demonstrate Tai Chi at an open house for the Shi-ho Center in Del Mar, CA. As he began his "moving meditation," the audience fell quiet and transfixed; the entire group went into a meditative state. Tsao allowed us to experience his radiating field of "Chi" (life force energy). Following this initial introduction to Tai Chi, I began studying with Master Tsao. I've since come to appreciate his remarkable skills and ability to communicate this ancient science and art to students at all levels of experience.

In recent years, there has been a dramatic increase in research dedicated to complementary and alternative medicine, which includes mind-body medicine, energy medicine, the use of prayer in healing, and the field of psychoneuroimmunology (PNI), the scientific field that investigates connections between stress, emotions, brain, and the immune system, and the implications of these linkages for health and disease. Western medicine now accepts the traditional Chinese belief that illness indicates an energy imbalance, and that health is best maintained by a balanced unimpeded flow of Chi.

Extensive scientific and empirical research in China has addressed the significant health benefits gained from regular Tai Chi practice for people with asthma, high blood pressure, circulatory and digestive problems, arthritis, in addition to complementing treatments for cancer, enhancing immune system functioning, improving balance, promoting emotional health and slowing the aging process. Western medicine has begun to research these areas and is already documenting some similar measures.

The cutting edge health care professionals of the new millennium will incorporate the ancient wisdom and teachings of mind-body approaches, like Tai Chi, along with Western technological advances to provide a truly holistic model of wellness promotion and health care.

Tsao's fundamental Compact Tai Chi is much more than a form of exercise. It is a self-healing approach that enhances and maintains health, and prevents disease by balancing body, mind, and spirit. Through his extensive experience teaching Tai Chi for wellness and stress management in the workplace—he taught superior court judges, attorneys, health care professionals, senior citizens and the general public, Tsao found he didn't have enough space! This lack of space resulted in a new integrated Tai Chi form—Compact Tai Chi!

The word "Master" is often over-used today. The true Master of any discipline must be able to communicate the basics to beginners. He must have the skill and knowledge to convey complexity to advanced students. In addition to being a great practitioner, he must be able to effectively pass down the traditions, philosophy and greater Truths. Master Tsao is a Master!

—KERRY J. KLUNER, M. D., FRCPC, Medical Director,
The Shi-ho Center for Creative & Healing Arts, Del Mar, CA

Acknowledgments

This book is dedicated to my wife—Julia Z. Tsao. Without her encouragement and support, this book would not have been possible.

I extend my special thanks to Mr. Joe Norris, who edited the first draft of this book, and Mr. Dan Bjerk, who proofread the first draft. Both of them are my long-time students. My great appreciation also goes to my friends Mr. Wei Yu and Mr. Jonathan Cong, who assisted me in setting up computer programs for loading photo images.

I also wish to thank Ms. Alexis Gordon, Ms. Cindy Gockel, and Mr. Murry Walker at the State of Arizona Employee Wellness office. They have facilitated hundreds of Tai Chi classes for me since 1994. They gave me the opportunity to teach Tai Chi as a work-site wellness program and, later, inspired me to invent the Spaceless Mini Tai Chi form.

Thanks to Mr. Mark Johannsson, Mr. Grant Piotti, and Mr. Kevin Montijo at PJRR Health Promotion System & Consulting firm. They encouraged me to apply Tai Chi in the field of complementary and alternative medicine, and in senior wellness programs.

I also wish to express my gratitude to Dr. Eric Monk, who sponsored me at the University of Arizona for my graduate study. Without him, I would not have been able to come to the United States and to do what I now love to do.

I would like to take this opportunity to thank Grand Master Deyin Li. He is the Vice Chairman of the Beijing Wushu Association and the Tai Chi drillmaster of the Chinese National Wushu team. I was fortunate to be his favorite student for over ten years, and to receive extensive special training from him in Beijing, China.

An Introduction to Compact Tai Chi

Tai Chi is an integrated exercise for the body, mind, and spirit. It improves physical characteristics such as flexibility, strength, balance, endurance, agility, and coordination. It relaxes the mind and helps it to deal effectively with the stress of modern living. It helps us to stay calm, alert and optimistic throughout our lives.

Tai Chi exercise relaxes our bodies and replenishes, rather than consumes, our energies. Numerous controlled studies conducted in China have shown that Tai Chi promotes healing and overall health, both physically and mentally. It not only strengthens the body and mind, but also has many positive effects on the immune system. In its country of origin, China, Tai Chi has been used extensively in many hospitals, where patients are taught to use Tai Chi to help them cure symptoms or speed recovery.

I have been teaching Tai Chi for over fourteen years in the United States. Hundreds of my students have enjoyed and benefited from Tai Chi. It is difficult, however, for most of them to find enough space in their homes or offices to practice the entire traditional Tai Chi form. This problem has become more apparent to me during the last several years, as I have taught Tai Chi to state employees in Arizona as a work-site wellness program. All the traditional Tai Chi forms require more room than is normally available at most work-sites. In response to this dilemma, I created the Spaceless Mini Tai Chi form, a form of the ancient art that requires minimal space. The new form takes only three to five minutes and requires less than 40 square feet of space. People can practice it right in front of their desks!

The success of the Spaceless Mini Tai Chi form inspired me to extend the idea into an innovative, comprehensive long form. Countless hours of research and many sleepless nights, combined with my more than 30 years of Tai Chi experience, have resulted in this multi-style, compact Tai Chi book. I hope this book makes Tai Chi much easier to practice in almost any location. I also hope it addresses the Tai Chi lovers' taste for different styles and combines the best aspects of each into one unique combined form.

There are four outstanding features of this book that distinguish it from traditional Tai Chi. These features make this book unique and user friendly to practitioners at all levels of expertise.

Clock Dial Format

One of the difficulties in learning Tai Chi from a book is that people get confused trying to follow directions for all the complex movements. This book attempts to solve this problem by using the face of the clock as a "map" for charting Tai Chi movements. This twelve-hour "map" gives you a clear, precise, and easy-to-follow reference for the movements for the whole form.

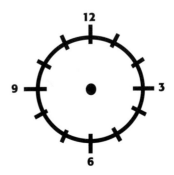

Compact Movements for Practicing in a Small Space

Compact Tai Chi is condensed to take only 25 to 30 percent of the practice space required for traditional Tai Chi. It is designed to fold and coil the traditional linear form into a more circular format. For example, the posture "Wave Hands Like Clouds" requires 3 to 5 steps to one side in the traditional form. It requires only one step in the coiling movement of the compact Tai Chi. The new form fits almost anywhere: the living room, patio, office, or even a small hotel room.

Combined Multi-Styles

Compact Tai Chi is designed to combine the five major Tai Chi styles into one comprehensive form. You can study all the different approaches in just one book. The five most popular Tai Chi styles in China are Yang, Chen, Wu, W'u, and Sun. The Chen style is the oldest, resembling the better-known martial arts, such as Kung Fu. The Yang style is the most popular style in America. It is less martial and demands less athleticism than the Chen. The Wu, W'u, and Sun styles were developed directly or indirectly from the Yang.

The new compact Tai Chi form is based largely on the Yang style. However, all repeated movements are deleted. The sequence begins with simple, easy-to-learn Yang movements and gradually adds movements from the Sun, Wu', and Chen styles. This new form is also more symmetrical, with a balance of left and right motion. To make the form more flexible and variable, it uses both the Yang style's vertical hand-circle transitions and the Wu and Sun style's horizontal hand-circle transitions. By adding the stepping techniques from the Sun style, this new form also increases agility and quickness. Finally, some fast movements from the Chen style are included for martial arts power.

Combined Multi-Levels

Unlike most traditional Tai Chi manuals, this book includes a set of four independent sequences to satisfy different levels of expertise and different practice schedules. You may practice the complete form or select one or two sequences, according to your physical strength and available time.

The first sequence is very easy to learn and practice. I call it "Tai Chi 101." It is especially designed for beginners, those who are not athletic, or those who have physical limitations. The sequence covers twelve postures and requires little space and time to practice. It is also useful as a workplace stress reducer and energy enhancer. It starts with the basic and simple postures, such as "Part Wild Horse's Mane" and "White Crane Spreads Its Wings." These two postures emphasize the fundamental principle of coordinating your torso and four limbs, as well as the shifting of your body weight.

The second sequence ("Tai Chi 201") is designed to improve flexibility, strength, balance, agility, and coordination, as well as to increase the range of motion in your arms, legs, and torso. After finishing this sequence, you will feel increased physical fitness, more energy, and greater strength.

The third and fourth sequences ("Tai Chi 301" and "Tai Chi 401") are designed for advanced practitioners. They offer more challenges because they include elements from the Chen, Sun, and Wu styles. By mastering all four sequences, you can gain a new and exhilarating understanding of Tai Chi and profit greatly from its practice.

I have used several new techniques to make this new form easier for you to learn. Each posture is illustrated with an average of six photos to show each movement in detail. Arrows indicate the direction of each foot and hand movement. The photos help you to learn the basic movements; the descriptions that accompany them are intended to help you better understand the finer details. Key Points are added after the movement descriptions to help you better understand the movements. Most of the Key Points remind you to keep the body and limbs relaxed and in good alignment. A Self-Defense Application is also included for each posture for those who love the martial arts. They are intended to show that Tai Chi is more than just a slow dance or a passive exercise.

The slow motions of Tai Chi may seem relatively simple, yet coordinating the numerous body movements into one integrated movement is not as easy as it may appear. This book contains four independent sequences, starting with the most basic and simple postures. Each section includes an optional closing posture. The first sequence places emphasis on fundamental techniques: the coordination of your torso and four limbs, as well as the correct shifting of body weight and proper foot movement. This sequence is easy to learn and is suitable for anyone of any age, regardless of athletic ability. Repeated practice of this short sequence will result in the comfortable coordination of the whole body. It will help build a solid foundation for further study. After mastering each sequence, you can move on to the next, more challenging one. With diligent practice, almost anyone can master the entire compact Tai Chi form.

GENERAL CHARACTERISTICS AND KEY GUIDELINES

Soft and Gentle

Tai Chi emphasizes the cultivation of internal energy. The movements should be performed in a sequence of smooth, slow, and steady manner. Tai Chi does not rely on brute strength. Rather, its tremendous power derives from the apparent gentleness of its movements. This external softness, however, conceals an internal hardness. It is a pliable strength rather than a tensed strength. It is "the steel wrapped in cotton."

Proper Body Alignment

Proper body alignment is essential to Tai Chi. Your head should be upright and your neck relaxed. Imagine that a wire suspends your head from above. Keep your body centered and upright. Keep your chest curved in and your back rounded up. Keep your waist and hips loose. Drop your shoulders and lower your elbows to loosen your shoulder joints. Adjust your body structure to sense the downward pull of gravity from body weight.

Wholeness and Harmony

There are nine major joints in your body: waist, hips, spine, shoulders, neck, elbows, wrists, knees, and ankles. Integrate these major joints into one motion. Coordinate your upper and lower body, as well as your mind. When one part of your body moves, all the other parts also move.

Your waist should always play the dominant role, since it connects your upper and your lower body. Once your waist moves, the other joints in the body should follow. Make your body pivot on your waist.

Maintain a Low Center of Gravity

Root your feet to the ground for a solid and firm stance. Bend your knees slightly and loosen your waist and hips. Maintain a low center of gravity to relax your upper body. Loosen your neck, spine, shoulders, and elbows for an unimpeded flow of inner energy. By doing so, you will wash stress and tension down through your feet into the ground. When stepping, shift your weight gradually from one leg to the other. Always remain aware of your center of gravity. Let your movements flow; don't bob up and down.

Abdominal Breathing

Maintain a natural breathing pattern. Do not force yourself to follow an artificial pattern. Find your own rhythm of inhalation and exhalation. Tai Chi promotes deep and slow abdominal breathing because of its slow and gentle movements. Abdominal breathing makes you more relaxed and your breathing more efficient.

As your movements become smooth, you can coordinate your breathing with your body movements. Normally, you inhale while your hands or arms go backward or inward (toward your body), and exhale while they go forward or outward (away from your body). When your arms move in opposite directions, your breathing should follow the major action arm (the arm making the larger or more important movement).

Concentration and Regulating Energy Flow through the Mind

Your mind leads the movements of your body and provides guidance for the inner energy flow. Try to sense this and lead the inner energy to specific areas of your body, integrating it with your physical movements. You can also use your mind to achieve balance, transferring the energy from areas where there is too much to those with too little. Normally, you should keep your mind focused on your lower abdomen (the "Dan Tian") to prevent the scattering of your thoughts and inner energy. When you pay attention to your abdominal breathing, your body stimulates your kidneys to produce more energy to nourish your body.

Circularity and Rotation

Just as nature abhors a vacuum, Tai Chi abhors a straight line. Your arms should always be curved and should move in circular patterns. Do not lock your elbows. Your arms should follow the movement of your waist. Circular movement is a natural extension of the spine and the rotary nature of bones, joints, and ligaments. Your arms should always be rotating when they move. The rotary aspect of Tai Chi is best demonstrated by the constant turning in and out of your palms during exercise. As an extra benefit, this non-stop circular motion of your arms effectively massages your shoulders, elbows, and wrists.

Weight Shifting, and Fullness and Emptiness in Steps

Your body weight usually concentrates on one leg during practice. The leg that bears the most weight is called the "full leg"; the other is called the "empty leg." The full leg implies firmness and stability. The empty leg implies the ability to change. While practicing the forms, your weight should constantly shift from one leg to the other. You cannot maintain stability or move skillfully without shifting your weight appropriately.

Fundamental Techniques

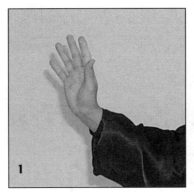

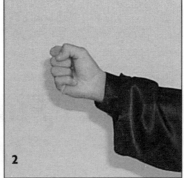

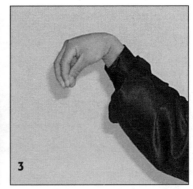

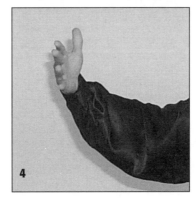

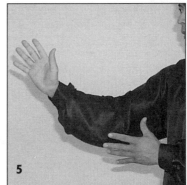

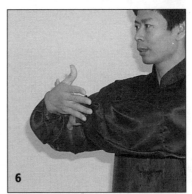

Hands and Arms

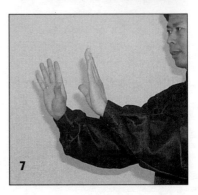

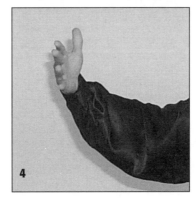

Open Palm (Figure 1)

This is the most common hand position in Tai Chi. Your fingers should be spaced naturally and extended slightly. Your palm should be rounded and full of energy. When you push out your palm, flex your wrist by extending the base of your palm forward, leaving your fingertips suspended in place. The small setting movement of your wrist can increase the penetrating power of your palm's strike.

Fist (Figure 2)

The fist is formed by folding your fingers and placing your thumb on the outside of the second section of your index and middle fingers. Hold your fist with your fingers lightly clenched in a tight grip.

Hook (Figure 3)

Bend your wrist slightly down and bring your fingertips and thumb together.

Ward Off (Figure 4)

This is the most common arm movement in Tai Chi. Curve your forearm slightly and raise it upward and forward to shoulder level, palm facing your chest. Use your mind to lead the energy flow to the outside of your forearm—the striking surface. This arm movement can be used to ward off blows from above, the front, or the side.

Roll Back (Figure 5)

Keep your arms rounded and your palms facing each other, diagonally. As you turn your upper body, move your palms down and back in a curve. The energy flowing from your palms makes it easier to grab and hold an opponent.

Press (Figure 6)

Place one palm on the inside of your opposite wrist and extend both hands forward at shoulder level. Keep both arms rounded and firm. Your mind leads the energy flow to the leading forearm and into your fingers.

Push (Figure 7)

This is a common Tai Chi hand movement. With your palms facing outward, push them in a forward and upward curve. Keep both elbows bent slightly, so that your arms curve upward. Do not allow your wrists to go higher than your shoulders. As you push forward, shift your weight forward and bend your front knee slightly.

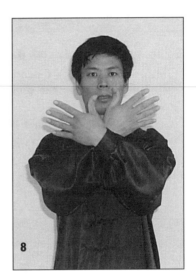

8

Cross Hands (Figure 8)

Cross your hands at the wrist in front of your chest, with palms facing inward. Keep both your arms in a curved shape.

Forward Punch (Figure 9)

Hold your fist at your side at waist level, with the "fist eye" (formed by the index finger and thumb) facing outward. As you punch the fist out from your waist, rotate your hand inward, turning your fist so that the fist eye faces up.

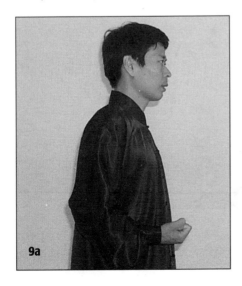

9a

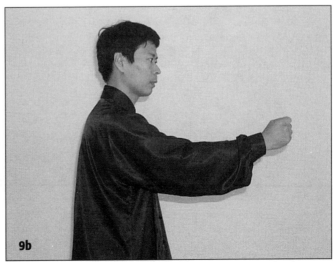

9b

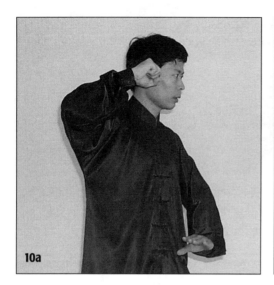

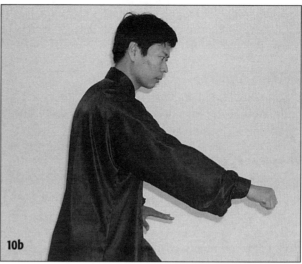

Downward Punch (Figure 10)

The downward punch begins at the side of your ear and moves down in front of your body, with the back of your fist facing up and the fist eye facing inward.

Ears Punch (Figure 11)

The ears punch starts at your lower waist, with both fist eyes facing outward. As you bring your fists up in curves from both sides of your body to ear height, rotate them so that your fist eyes face diagonally downward. Keep your shoulders relaxed, elbows dropped, and arms rounded.

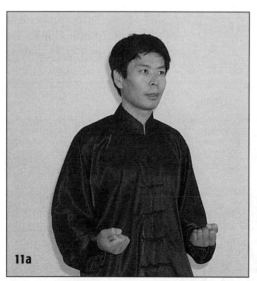

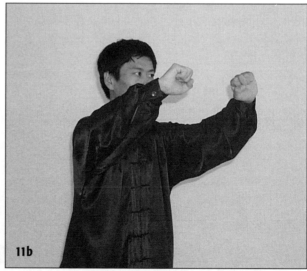

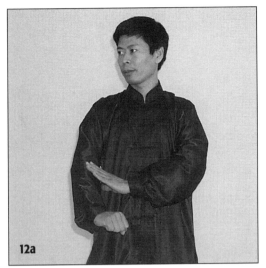

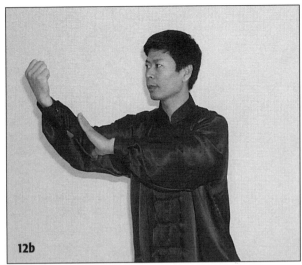

Back of Fist Punch (Figure 12)

Hold your right fist in front of the left side of your abdomen, with the back of your fist facing out. Curve your left palm above your right forearm, palm facing downward. Then, turn your body to the right and bring your right fist across your face in a circular motion, punching forward at face level. As you punch out, rotate your fist so that the back of the fist is leading. Place your left hand inside the forearm of your punching hand to reinforce the punch and protect the punching arm's elbow.

Palm Spear Up (Figure 13)

In this movement, the palm starts low and moves in a curve to spear up in front of your body to face level, fingers facing up.

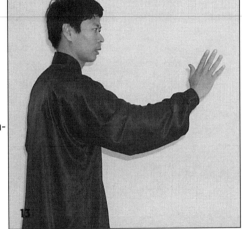

Palm Spear Down (Figure 14)

In this movement, the palm starts high and moves diagonally down in front of your body to waist level, fingers facing diagonally downward.

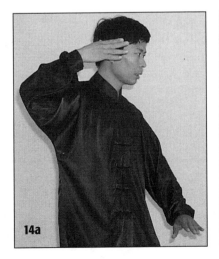

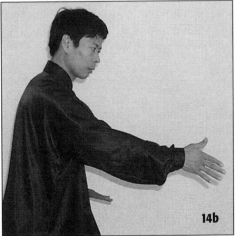

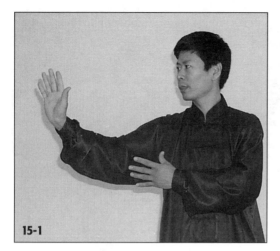

15-1

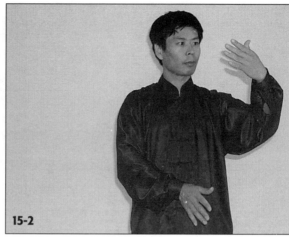

15-2

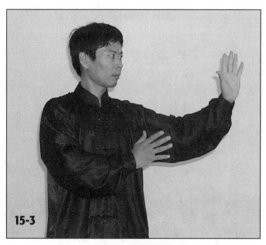

15-3

Wave Hand (Figure 15)

1. Turn your body slightly to the right, and move your left palm in front of your right shoulder, with the palm facing obliquely inward. Simultaneously, push your right hand toward the right, fingers pointing up. Keep both arms curved and both elbows dropped.

2. Turning your body toward the left, move your left hand up and to the left in a curve, passing your face. Simultaneously, move your right hand in a downward circle past your abdomen.

3. Continue turning your body to the left and rotate your left palm out and to the left side of your body, palm facing out. At the same time, bring up your right palm in a circular motion to the front of your left shoulder, the palm slowly turning inward.

Holding the Ball (Figure 16)

Hold your palms facing each other in front of your chest, as though you were holding a beach ball. Your upper hand should be at shoulder level and your lower hand at your waist. Keep both elbows relaxed and your arms rounded.

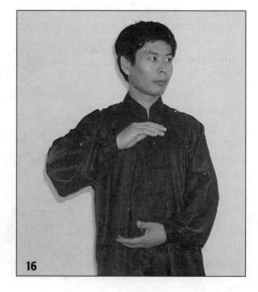

16

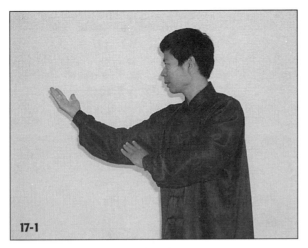

17-1

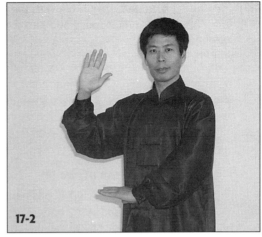

17-2

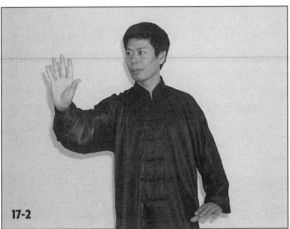

17-2

Block Down and Push (Figure 17)

1. Turn your body to the right. Block your left hand down in front of your right chest and bring your right hand up from behind in a circular motion to ear level, keeping your arm slightly bent and your palm facing obliquely upward.

2. Turn your body to the front, curving your right forearm. Push your right palm forward by the side of your right ear at nose level, with the palm facing forward. At the same time, block down your left forearm and pull your left palm to the side of your left hip, with fingers pointing forward.

3. Turn your body to the left and move your right hand in a curve to the front of your left chest with the palm facing down. Bring your left hand up from behind (in a circular motion) to ear level, with your arm bending slightly and your palm facing obliquely upward.

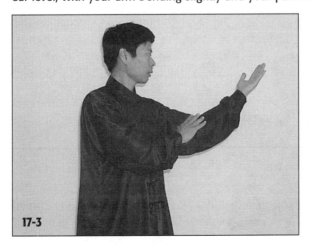

17-3

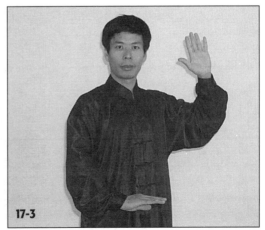

17-3

11

4. Repeat Step 2, but with the opposite hands blocking and pushing.

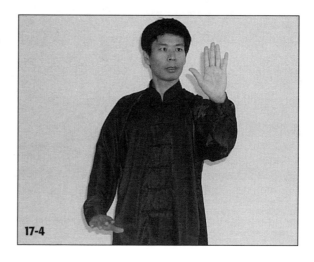

Block Up and Push (Figure 18)

1. From a holding-ball position, with your left hand at the bottom, turn your body slightly to the left, and move your left hand up across your chest and face to the left side of your forehead, your left palm rotating obliquely upward. At the same time, move your right hand in a small downward curve before pushing it up and forward to nose level, fingers pointing up.

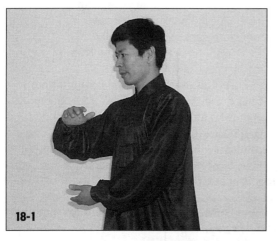

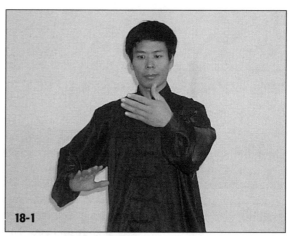

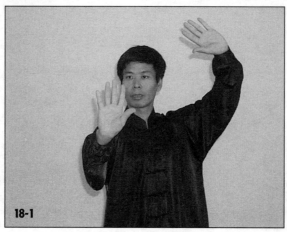

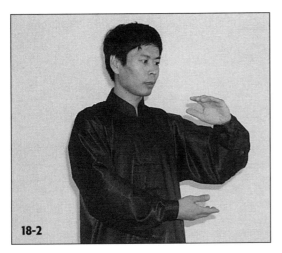

18-2

2. Form a holding-ball posture by moving your right hand in a downward curve at waist level with the palm turning up, and moving your left hand down to shoulder level with the palm turning down.

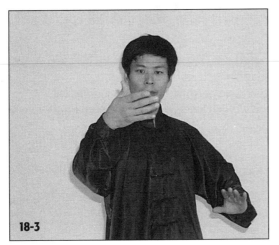

18-3

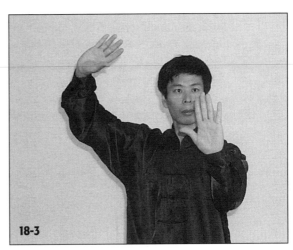

18-3

3. Repeat Step 1, but with the opposite hands blocking and pushing.

Stances

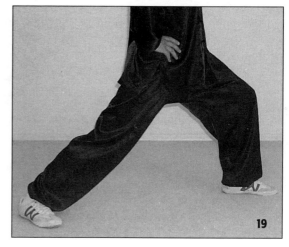

19

Bow Stance (Figure 19)

This is the most common stance in the Tai Chi exercise. Bend your front leg so that it resembles a bow being pulled. Do not extend your bent knee beyond your toes. The toes of your front foot point forward. Keep your back leg straight, but don't lock your knee. The toes of your back foot point diagonally forward by pivoting your heel slightly out. Do not place both feet in a straight line. Keep your feet a transverse distance of 12 inches.

Empty Stance (Figure 20)

Put your entire weight on your rear leg and squat down slightly, keeping your front leg "empty." The toes or heel of your front foot should touch the floor when your leg is completely relaxed. The empty leg implies the ability to change.

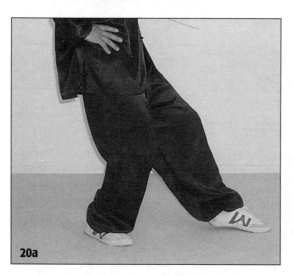

20a

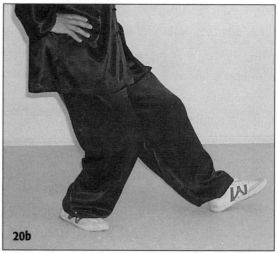

20b

Snake Creeps Down (Figure 21)

Squat down on one leg, keeping the other leg straight out and close to the ground with the toes turned inward. Keep both feet fully on the floor. Try to keep your body upright. Do not lean forward in order to get down a few inches farther. Your bent knee should point in the same direction as the toes of that foot to prevent your knee from being twisted. Squat down as low as you can without discomfort.

Resting Stance (Figure 22)

Cross your legs and squat down half way. The knee of your rear leg should be behind the calf of your front leg. Your entire front foot should touch the floor, while only the sole of your rear foot touches the floor. You can sink your body down totally to form a Lower Resting Stance.

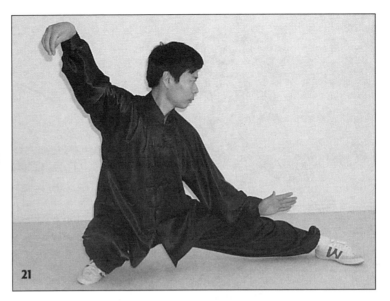

21

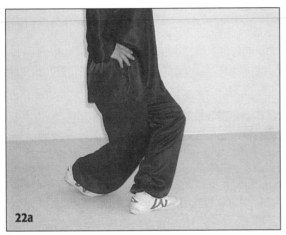

22a

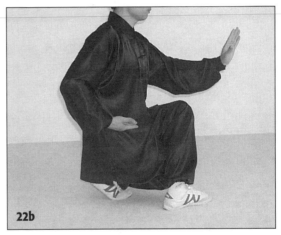

22b

Golden Rooster (Figure 23)

Stand straight up on one leg without locking your knee and lift your other knee as high as you can with the toes pointing down. Lower your center of gravity and root your standing leg deeply into the ground. This is a balance training.

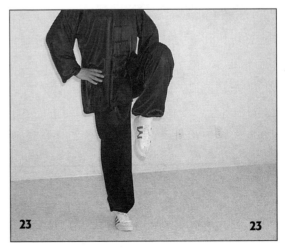

23   23

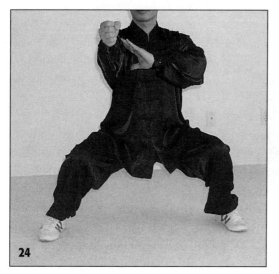

24

Horse-Riding Stance (Figure 24)

Stand with both feet about two shoulder-widths apart, toes pointing forward and slightly out. Bend both knees, but keep your back straight and vertical. Distribute your body weight evenly on both feet. When squatting down, do not bend your knees beyond your toes. Point your knees in the same direction as your feet.

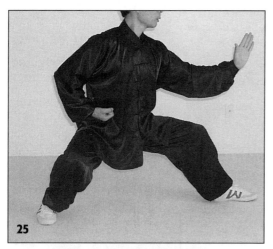

25

Half Horse-Riding Stance (Figure 25)

Stand with both feet about two shoulder-widths apart. Point your front toes forward and your back toes to the side. Bend both knees, keeping your back straight. Your back leg bears more body weight than your front leg. Keep your knees pointing in the same direction as your feet.

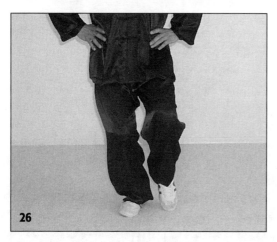

26

T-Stance (Figure 26)

Stand on one leg with the knee bent slightly and with all your weight on it. Place your empty foot next to the supporting foot, about four inches apart, with your toes touching the floor.

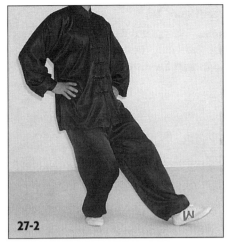

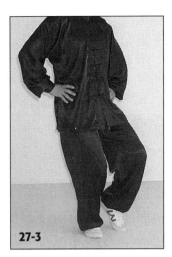

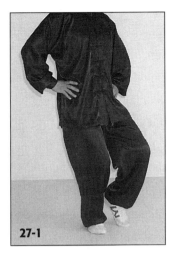

27-1

27-2

27-3

Stepping Forward (Figure 27)

1. Bend both knees and squat down slightly. Shift your weight to your right leg and lift your left foot heel, leaving your left toes touching the floor. Turn your head slightly to the left.

2. Step your left foot forward, letting your left heel touch the floor gently. Keep your right leg slightly bent and your left leg straight, but without locking your knee.

3. Pull back your left foot gently, placing it next to your right foot, with toes barely touching the floor.

4. Repeat Steps 2 and 3 three to five times. Then, pull back and step down on your left heel, shifting your body weight to your left leg. Do the same motions with your right foot.

Stepping and kicking

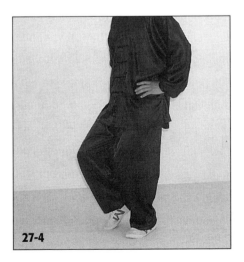

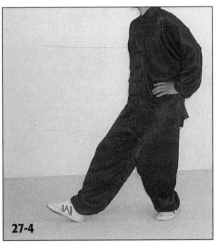

27-4

27-4

Walking in Tai Chi Step (Figure 28)

1. Bend both knees and squat down slightly. Shift your weight to your right leg. Turn your chest to the left and bring your left foot to your left, with the empty heel touching the floor first.

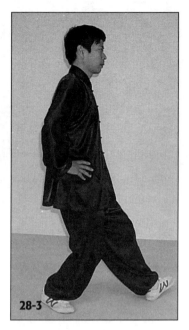

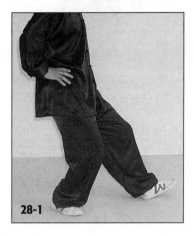

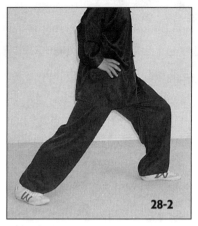

28-1

28-2

28-3

2. As you shift your weight forward, lower the sole of your left foot to the floor. Adjust your right foot in the back by pivoting your heel slightly out. Straighten your back knee without locking it. Bend your front knee, keeping knee and toes in alignment. Make sure your front knee does not extend beyond your toes.

3. Shift your weight back to your right leg. Lift up your left toes and rotate them outward slightly, while turning your body slightly to the left.

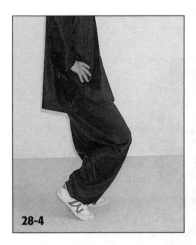

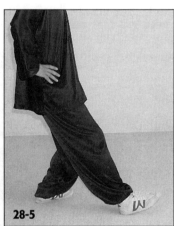

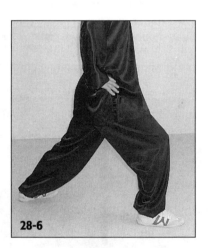

28-4

28-5

28-6

4. Move your body forward and lower the sole of your left foot to the floor. Shift your weight onto your left leg, bending that knee slightly. At the same time, bring your right foot next to your left foot with its toes barely touching the floor.

5. Step your right foot forward with your empty heel touching the floor first.

6. Repeat Step 2, but using the opposite foot.

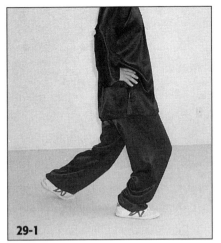

29-1

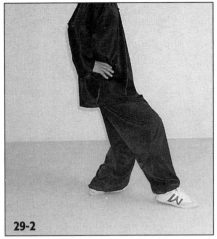

29-2

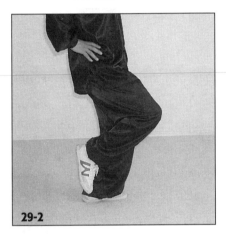

29-2

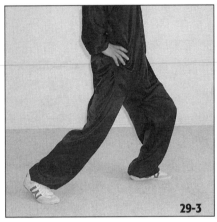

29-3

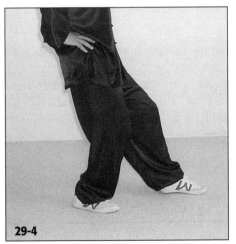

29-4

Stepping Backward (Figure 29)

1. Bend both knees and squat down slightly. Shift your weight to your right leg. Step backward with your left toes touching the floor first.

2. Shift your weight back onto your left leg and press down your left heel. After stepping back, adjust your front foot to an empty stance by lifting the heel off the floor.

3. Bring your right foot back, with the toes touching the floor first.

4. Repeat Step 2, but using the opposite foot.

19

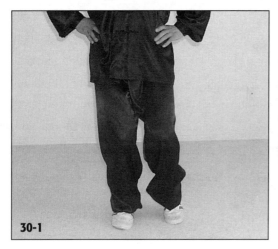

30-1

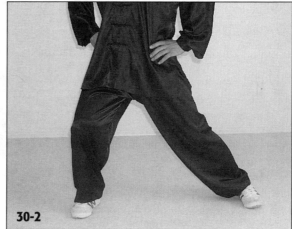

30-2

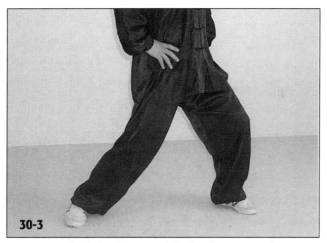

30-3

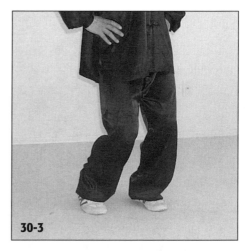

30-3

Side Stepping (Figure 30)

1. Bend both knees and squat down slightly. Shift your weight to your right leg. Lift up your left heel, with the toes barely touching the floor.

2. Turn your body to the right and step your left foot to the left, its toes touching the floor.

3. Turn your body to the left. Shift your weight to your left leg with your left heel pressing down. Bring your right foot closer to your left foot with both feet pointing forward. Keep your feet about 5–8 inches apart.

4. Shift your weight onto your right leg again, and repeat Steps 1, 2, and 3 again three to five times.

5. Repeat the side-stepping motion, but in the opposite direction.

Transforming Bow Stance by Pivoting Heels (Figure 31)

1. In a left bow stance, shift your weight onto your back leg and turn your body to the right. At the same time, lift your left toes and rotate them inward by pivoting on your left heel.

2. Shift your weight onto your left leg and continue turning your body to the right. Lift your right heel and bring your right foot next to your left, with toes touching the floor.

3. Continue turning your body to the right and step your right foot forward with the heel touching the floor first. Then, shift your weight forward to form a right bow stance.

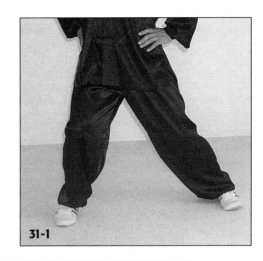

31-1

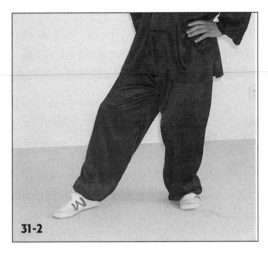

31-2

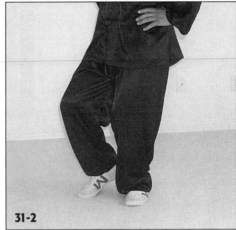

31-2

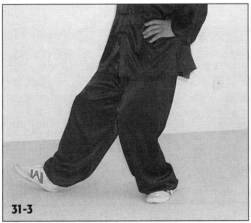

31-3

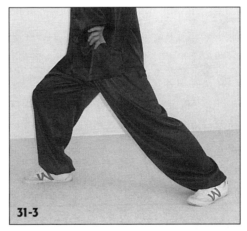

31-3

21

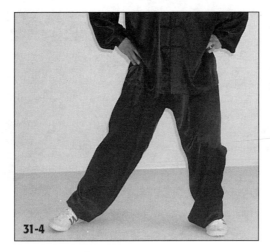

31-4

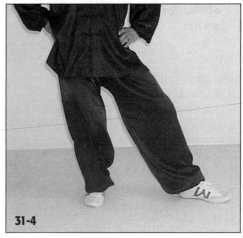

31-4

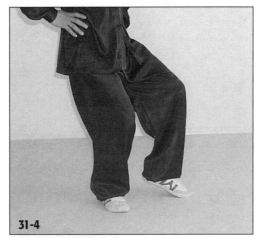

31-4

4. In a right bow stance, shift your weight onto your back leg and turn your body to the left. At the same time, lift your right toes and rotate them inward by pivoting on your right heel.

5. Shift your weight onto your right leg and continue turning your body to the left. Lift your left heel and bring your left foot next to your right, with toes touching the floor.

6. Continue turning your body to the left and step your left foot forward with the heel touching the floor first. Then, shift your weight forward to form a left bow stance.

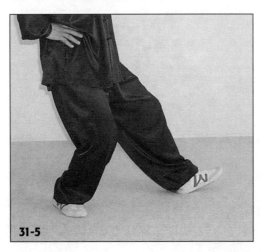

31-5

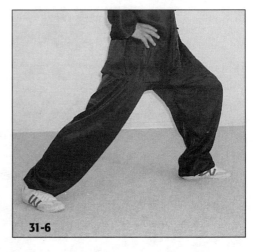

31-6

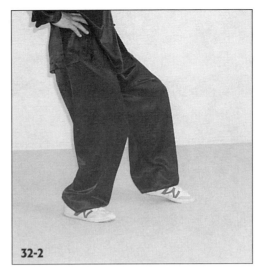

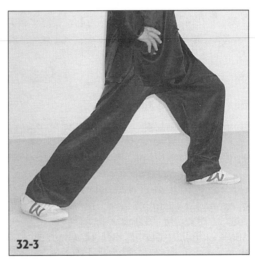

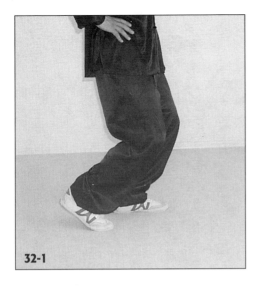

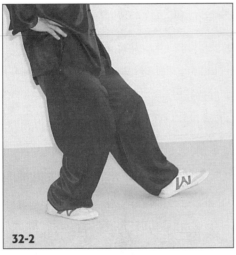

Half-Step Follow Up Stepping (Figure 32)

1. In a left bow stance, shift your weight forward and bring your back foot a half-step forward, behind your front heel, with the toes of your right foot touching the floor.

2. Shift your weight back to your right leg and press down your right heel. Meanwhile, lift your left heel and step your left foot forward, with the heel touching the floor.

3. Shift your weight forward. With your left sole press down, bend your left knee into a left bow stance.

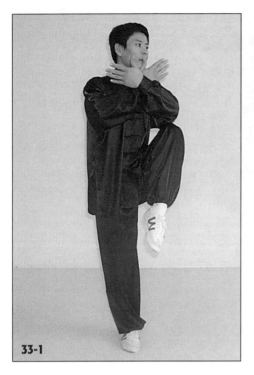

33-1

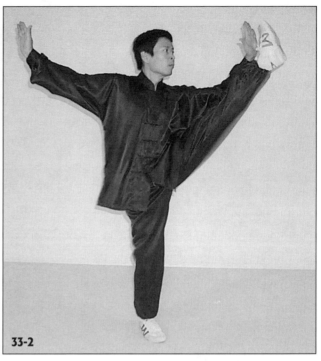

33-2

Heel Kick (Figure 33)

1. Stand on your right leg and lift your left knee. Cross your arms in front of your chest with palms facing inward.

2. Rotate and separate your palms, extending both arms with palms facing outward. Kick your left heel out, with your toes pointing up, so that your heel is the attacking point. Kick your left foot higher than waist level. Your left hand should be just above your left leg.

3. Bring your left foot back down. Shift your weight onto your left leg as you drop both hands and turn your body to the right.

4. Repeat Steps 1 and 2, but with your right heel kicking out.

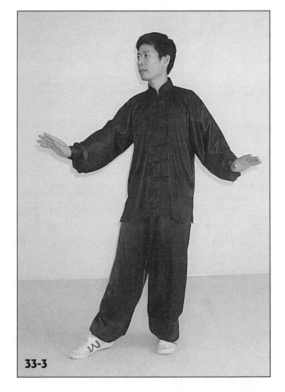

33-3

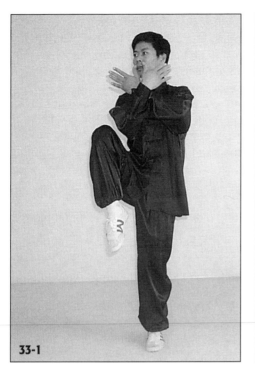

33-1

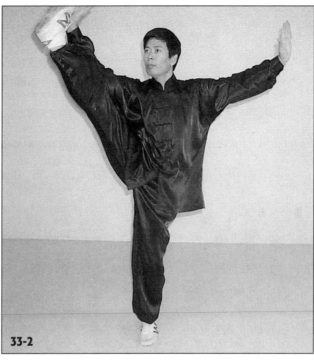

33-2

Toes Kick (Figure 34)

Repeat the steps used in the Heel Kick, but with your toes pointing outward as the attacking point.

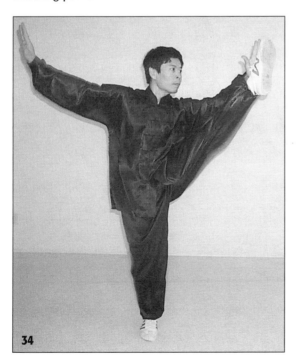

34

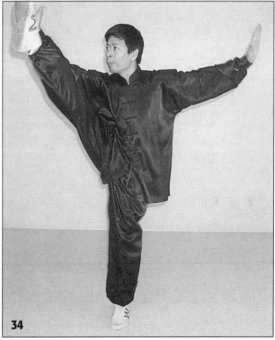

34

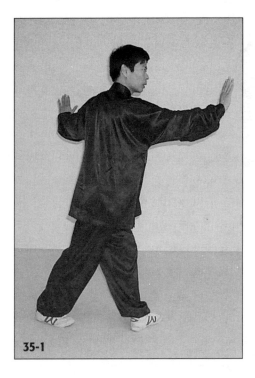

35-1

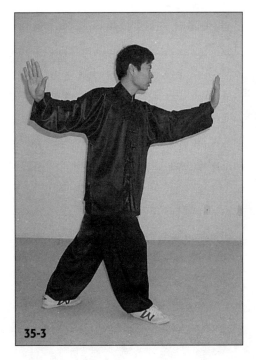

35-3

High Swing Kick and Slap Foot (Figure 35)

1. Step your left foot a half-step forward and shift your weight onto it. Raise both hands, with your left palm pushing backward to the left, and your right palm pushing forward at head level.

2. Straighten your left leg and swing kick your right foot to head height, with your instep stretched and flat. Make sure the instep of your right foot is the hitting point. At the same time, slap your right foot with your right palm.

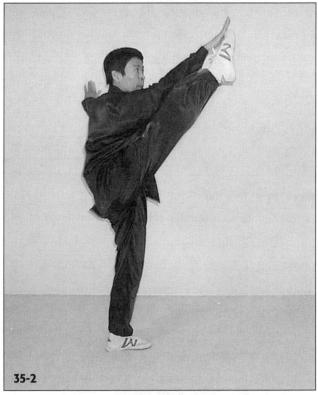

35-2

3. Step your right foot down in front of your body and shift your weight forward. At the same time, turn your chest to the right, circle your left palm up and forward, and circle your right palm down and back to your right rear.

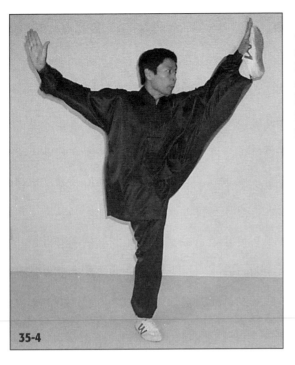

4. Repeat Step 2, but with the opposite foot and palm. Straighten your right leg and swing kick your left foot to head height, with your instep stretched and flat. Make sure the instep of your left foot is the hitting point. At the same time, slap your left foot with your left palm.

35-4

Side-to-Side Sweep Lotus Kick (Figure 36)

1. Shift your weight to your left leg and turn your body slightly to the left. At the same time, move both palms to your right side, with the right palm at face level and the left palm in front of your right chest.

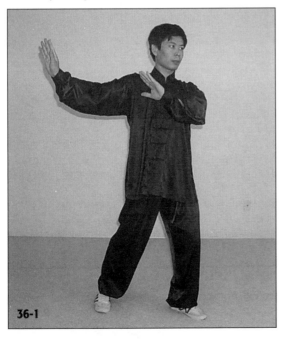

36-1

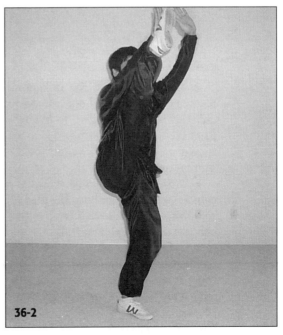

36-2

2. Sweep your right foot in a curve in front of you at face level. As the foot passes in front of your face, slap both palms across its instep. When you do so, keep the kicking-foot instep stretched and flat.

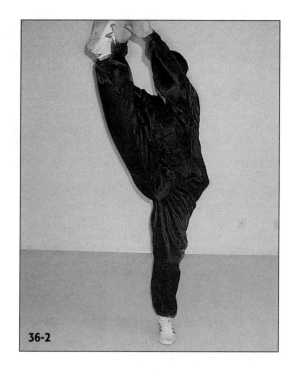

36-2

Power Emitting

Roll Back and Press Out (Figure 37)

1. Step your right foot back, move both hands to your left front with palms obliquely facing each other. Your left palm should be slightly up and forward at shoulder level. Your right palm should be next to your left elbow.

2. Shift your weight back to your right leg and turn your body slightly to your right. Roll both hands down to the front of your abdomen.

3. Turn your body to the left. Bring both hands up in a circular motion. Curve your left forearm across your chest with the left palm facing inward, while placing your right palm inside your left wrist. Stay

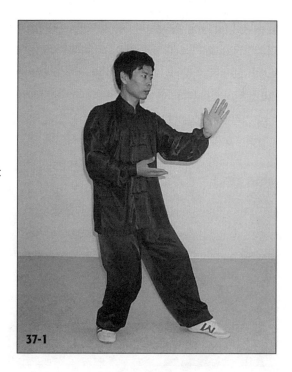

37-1

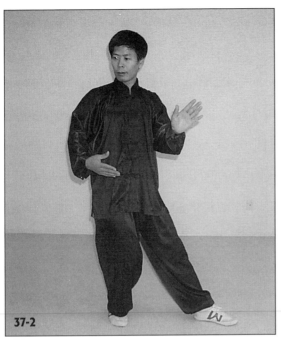

37-2

relaxed and store up power on your waist and back. Look to the front.

4. Press your right foot against the ground and push your body forward quickly, using the power in your waist and right leg. The internal power flows onto your arms to press out your left forearm with explosive force.

5. Repeat Steps 1 through 4, with the opposite arm pressing out.

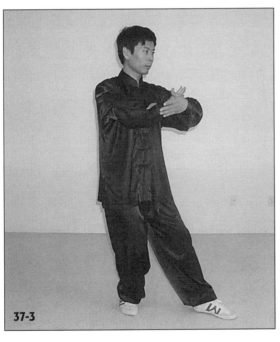

37-3

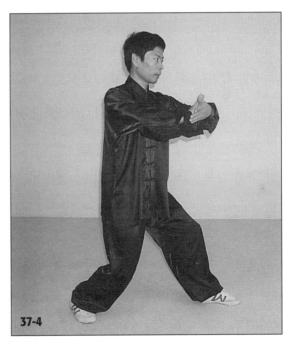

37-4

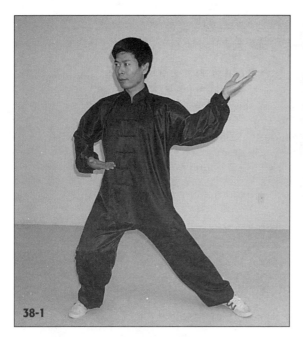

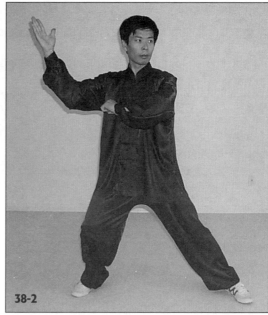

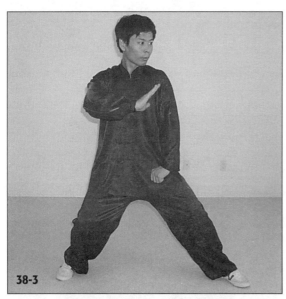

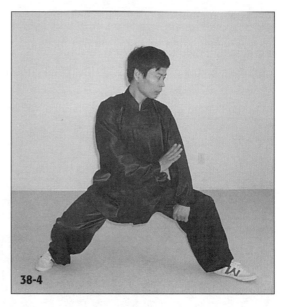

Press and Shoulder Stroke (Figure 38)

1. Step your right foot to the right and shift your weight to your right leg. Turn your body to the right slightly as you bring up your left hand at shoulder level, with palm facing up. At the same time, turn your right palm up to the right of your waist. Look to the right.

2. Move your left hand in a curve across your face, down to the front of your right chest, with the hand clenched into a fist. Move your right hand up from your right side with the palm facing obliquely to the left. Turn your head to look at your left side.

3. Move your right hand down in front of your left chest, with the palm facing to the left. Drop your left fist in front of your left thigh, with the fist eye facing inward. Breathe deeply and store up power on your waist and back. Look to the left.

4. Press your right foot against the ground and push your body to the left, quickly, by the power in your right leg and waist. Bend your left leg slightly into a half horse-riding stance. Press and stroke your left shoulder and upper arm to the left side, with the right palm closer to the inside of your left arm to enforce the stroke. Look to the left.

Power Punch (Figure 39)

1. Separate your feet to a distance of two shoulder-widths. Bring your hands up from both sides. Turn your body to the left and bend your left leg slightly, with your right leg straight.

2. Shift your weight and turn your body to the right, with your right leg bent slightly down. Lower both hands in a circular motion in front of your face, with your left palm turning up at shoulder level. Clench your right hand into a fist inside your left elbow, with the back of your hand facing downward. Breathe in deeply and store up power on your back. Look at your left palm.

3. Press your right foot against the ground and turn your body to the left,

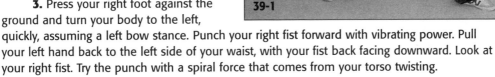

39-1

quickly, assuming a left bow stance. Punch your right fist forward with vibrating power. Pull your left hand back to the left side of your waist, with your fist back facing downward. Look at your right fist. Try the punch with a spiral force that comes from your torso twisting.

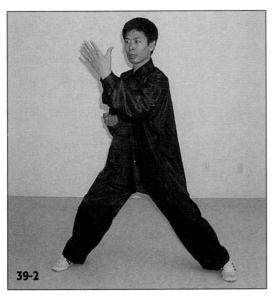

39-2

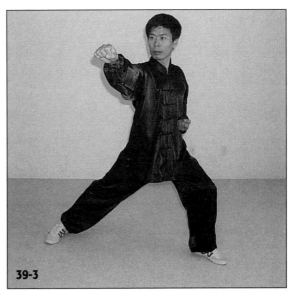

39-3

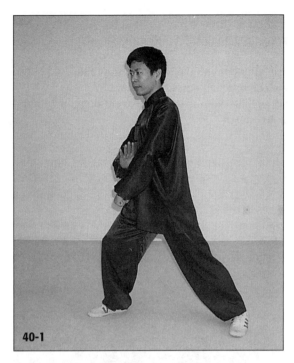

40-1

Throw Fist Aside (Figure 40)

1. Step your right foot to the right and shift your weight onto your right leg. Turn your body to the right slightly, as you clench your left hand into a fist and move it to the right side of your abdomen. At the same time, place your right palm inside your left forearm. Look to your right.

2. Move your left fist up to shoulder level, with your right palm following. Breathe in and store up power on your waist and back. Turn your head to the left.

3. Press your right foot against the ground and turn your body to the left, into a left bow stance. At the same time, throw your left fist to your left, quickly. The punching power comes from your right foot, through your waist and shoulder, to the back of your hand. Keep your right palm on the inside of your left forearm to enhance the power. Look at your left fist.

4. Repeat Steps 1 through 3 with the opposite arm.

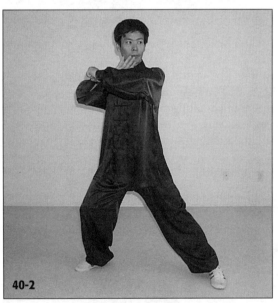

40-2

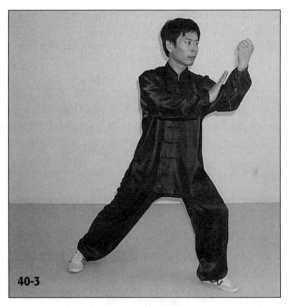

40-3

Sequence

1

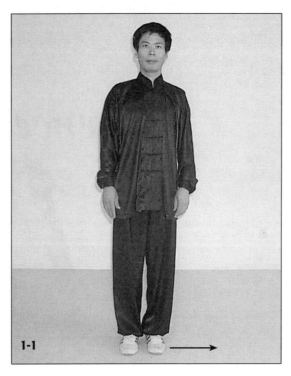

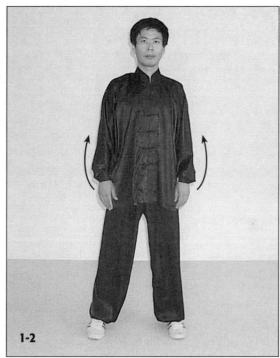

1-1

1-2

Posture 1

COMMENCING FORM

Imagine you are standing at the center of a big clock dial. You are facing 6 o'clock. Your back is at 12 o'clock. Your right side is at 9 o'clock. Your left side is at 3 o'clock.

Movement 1

Stand upright, with your body relaxed. Put your feet together and let your arms down. Breathe naturally, concentrate, and face forward.

Movement 2

Shift your weight to your right leg. Lift your left foot gently and place it to the left, about a shoulder-width from your right leg. Both feet should be parallel, with the toes pointing forward. Distribute your weight evenly on both legs. Hold your head and neck erect with your chin drawn slightly inward.

Movement 3

Raise your arms to the front slowly, to shoulder level, with the palms facing down. Keep your hands a shoulder-width apart.

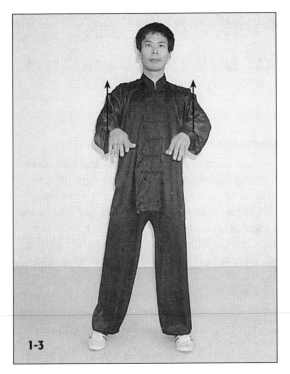

1-3

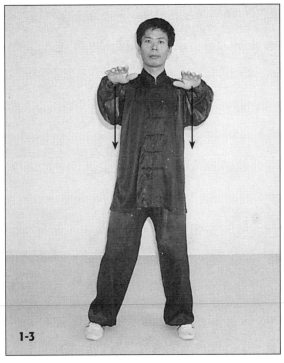

1-3

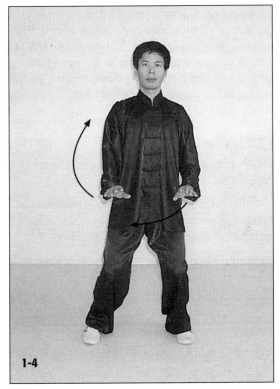

1-4

Movement 4

Bend your knees and squat slightly. Lower your arms, while pressing your palms down slowly. Look to the front.

☑ Key Points

1. Keep your body erect and relax your shoulders and elbows. Your hands and fingers should be curved naturally.

2. While bending your knees, keep your waist relaxed and your buttocks tucked in slightly.

3. The lowering of your arms should be coordinated with the bending of your knees. Keep your elbows low at all times.

4. Face 6 o'clock in the final position.

☑ Self-Defense Application

Intercept your attacker's arms by raising up your hands. Then, strike your attacker's chest by pressing your palm down and forward.

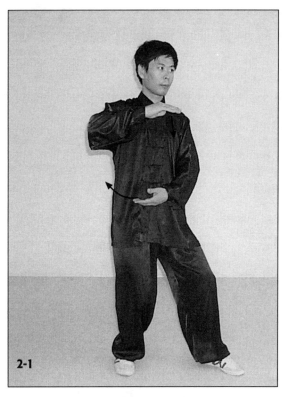

2-1

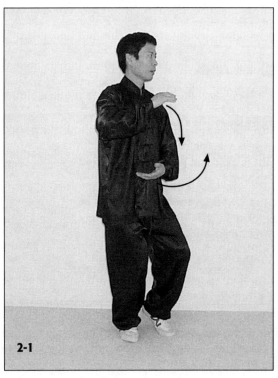

2-1

Posture 2

PART WILD HORSE'S MANE–LEFT

Movement 1

Turn your body slightly to the right and shift your weight to your right leg. Raise your right hand to the front of your right chest, with the palm facing down, while moving your left hand in a downward curve until it comes under your right hand. Your palms should be facing each other as if holding a ball. Bring your left foot to the side of your right foot, with its toes touching the floor. Look at your right hand.

Movement 2

Turn your body to the left to the 4 o'clock position. Step with your left foot toward a position midway between 2 and 3 o'clock. Bend your left knee and shift your weight onto your left leg to form a left bow stance. As your body turns left, raise your left hand to eye level with the palm facing obliquely up and pull your right hand down to the side of your right hip with the palm facing down and fingers pointing forward. Look at your left palm.

✅ Key Points

1. Hold your upper body erect and your chest relaxed. Keep your body straight.

2. Maintain your arms in a circular extension when separating your hands. Your back muscles should be stretched while your arms are extending.

3. Always pivot at the waist when turning your body.

4. Your movements as you take the bow stance and separate your hands should be smooth and synchronized.

5. When taking a bow stance, place your front foot in position slowly, with your heel coming down first. Do not bend your knees beyond the toes.

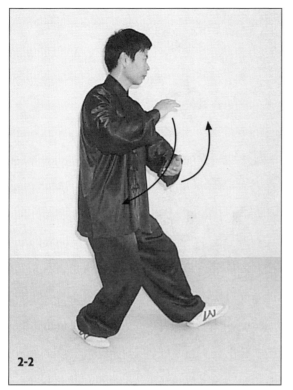

2-2

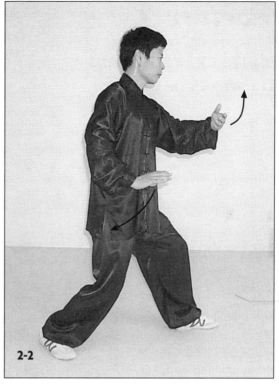

2-2

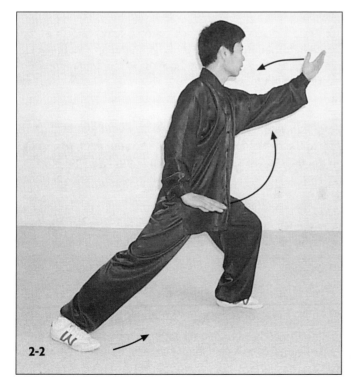

2-2

Keep your rear leg straight, but not locked.

6. There should be a transverse distance of 12 inches between your heels in order to keep a good balance and an easy energy flow.

7. Face 3 o'clock in the final position.

☑ Self-Defense Application

Intercept and grab your attacker's arm or hand to pull him down with your right hand, while moving your left forearm up and forward to your attacker's armpit to strike and control him. The striking power is energized by your waist, not just your left arm.

Posture 3

WHITE CRANE SPREADS ITS WINGS—LEFT

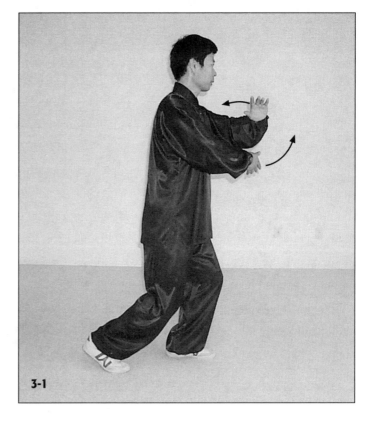

3-1

Movement 1

Turn your body slightly to the left, to the 2 o'clock position. Draw your left hand back in a curve in front of your chest with the palm turned down. Turn your right palm up and bring it across your waist in a curve to "hold a ball," with your left hand on top. At the same time, bring your right foot a half step toward your left foot.

Movement 2

Bring your right heel down and gently lean your upper body back, shifting your weight onto your right leg. Turn your body slightly to the right, to 4 o'clock, and move your left foot slightly forward, resting your toes lightly on the floor to form a left empty step. Both legs should be bent slightly at the knees.

Movement 3

As you turn your body slightly back to the left, to 3 o'clock, slowly raise your right hand in front of you, toward your right temple, with the palm turning outward. Move your left hand down to your left hip with your palm turning down and your fingers pointing forward. Look to the front.

✔ Key Points

1. Do not thrust your chest forward or raise your shoulders. Keep your elbows down.

2. As you shift your weight forward, this should be coordinated with placing your arms in the hold-ball position. As you shift your weight backward, you should simultaneously lower your left palm and raise your right palm.

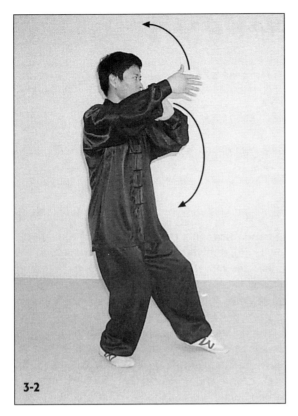

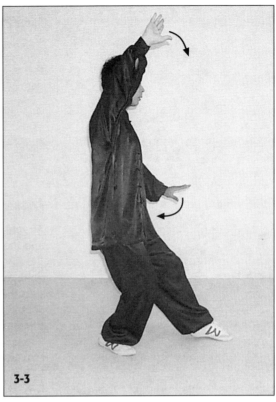

3-2

3-3

3. Round your arms when separating your hands. Prop up your right forearm and palm with flexible strength.

4. Face 3 o'clock in the final position.

☑ Self-Defense Application

Use your right hand and forearm to protect your head, chest, and upper right side from your attacker's punch. Use your left hand to block your abdomen and left hip, in case your attacker tries to kick your lower body. The motion is generated from the waist, not just the arms. The right arm moving up and spreading has the purpose of warding off a blow. In coordination with the arm motion, you can also kick your attacker's lower body with your left foot, since all your body weight is on your right leg.

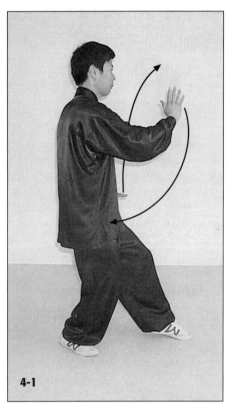

4-1

Posture 4

BRUSH KNEE—LEFT

Movement 1

As your right hand moves in a curve to the left of your chest and then downward, turn your body slightly to the left, to 2 o'clock, to lead the movement. Turn your body back to the right, to 4 o'clock, to bring your left hand up in a curve to your right chest. While your body turns right, your right hand should circle past your abdomen, then up to ear level, with the arm bending slightly and the palm facing obliquely upward. Your left hand should continue its circle in a right downward curve to the right side of your body, with the palm facing obliquely downward. Bring your left foot back, toes touching the floor.

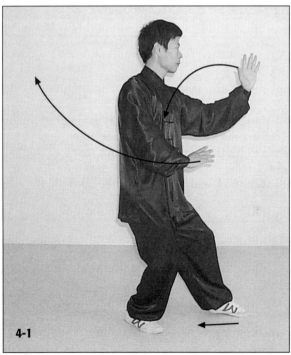

4-1

Movement 2

Turn your body to the left, to 3 o'clock, as you step your left foot to the 2 o'clock position to form a left bow stance. Shift your major weight onto your left leg. At the same time, curve your right forearm and push your right hand forward by the side of your right ear at nose level, with the palm facing forward. Bring your left hand down in a circular motion and brush past your left knee, coming to rest beside your left hip. Look at the fingertips of your right hand.

☑ Key Points

1. When your left foot steps out, push your right hand out as your body weight shifts forward. The right hand pushing depends more on the body movement than on the arm.

2. Keep a transverse distance of 12 inches between your heels in a bow stance to hold a firm balance and an easy energy flow.

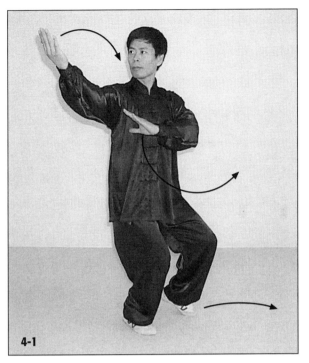

4-1

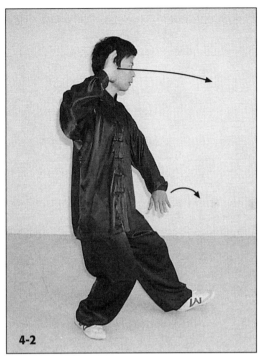

4-2

3. Keep your body erect. Drop your shoulder and keep your elbows down. Relax your waist and hips.

4. The left arm moves in a clockwise circle and the right arm moves in a counter-clockwise circle. Remember, your body's turn initiates your arm's motion.

5. Face 3 o'clock in the final position.

✓ Self-Defense Application

Block your attacker's punches by using your right arm, moving down and to the left, and your left arm, moving up and to the right. Both blocks are energized by your waist, not your arms. Following the two blocks, step your left foot forward to push your attacker with your right palm.

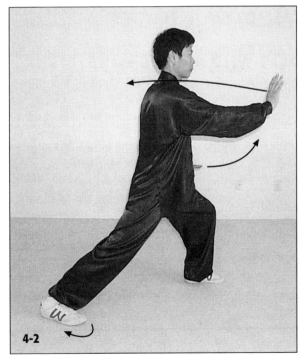

4-2

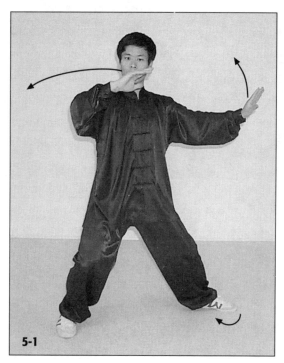
5-1

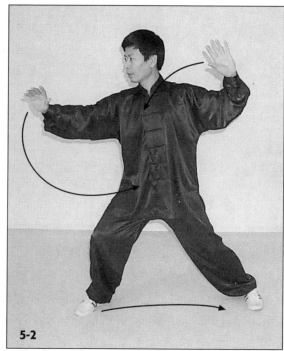
5-2

Posture 5

PART WILD HORSE'S MANE–RIGHT

Movement 1

Rotate your right toes outward slightly as you shift your body weight onto your right leg and turn your body to the right, to 7 o'clock. Rotate your left toes inward. Move your right hand in an arc to the right, with the palm turning downward and outward. Move your left hand up to shoulder level. Look at your right hand.

Movement 2

Shift your body weight back to your left leg and turn your body to the left, to 6 o'clock. Bring your right foot back to the side of your left foot, with the toes on the floor. At the same time, move your right hand down to rest below your left rib, and bring your left hand back to lie in front of your chest, with the palm facing down to form a hold-ball position.

Movement 3

Turn your body to the right, to the 8 o'clock position. Step with your right foot toward a position midway between 9 and 10 o'clock. Bend your right knee and shift your weight onto your right leg to form a right bow stance. As your body turns right, raise your right hand to eye level with the palm facing obliquely up and pull your left hand down to the side of your left hip with the palm facing down and fingers pointing forward. Look at your right palm.

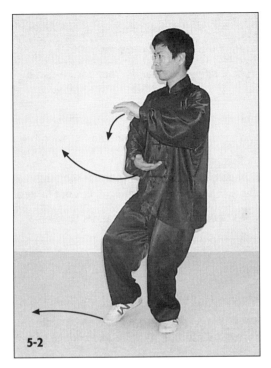

5-2

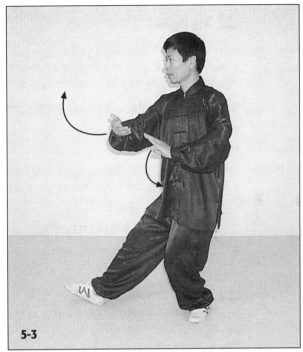

5-3

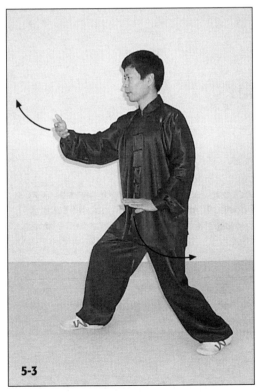

5-3

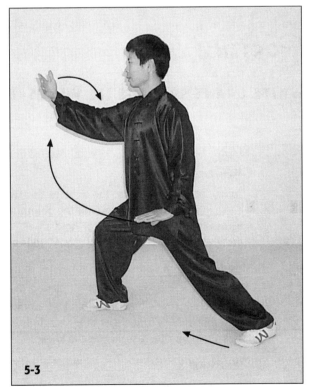

5-3

✅ Key Points

1. Hold your upper body erect and your chest relaxed. Keep your body straight.

2. Maintain your arms in a circular extension when separating your hands. Your back muscles should be stretched while your arms are extending.

3. Always pivot at the waist when turning your body.

4. Your movements as you take the bow stance and separate your hands should be smooth and synchronized.

5. When taking a bow stance, place your front foot in position slowly with your heel coming down first. Do not bend your knees beyond the toes. Keep your rear leg straight, but not locked.

6. There should be a transverse distance of 12 inches between your heels in order to keep a good balance and an easy energy flow.

7. Face 9 o'clock in the final position.

✅ Self-Defense Application

Intercept and grab your attacker's arm or hand to pull him down with your left hand, while moving your right forearm up and forward to your attacker's armpit to strike and control him. The striking power is energized by your waist, not just your right arm.

Posture 6

WHITE CRANE SPREADS ITS WINGS—RIGHT

Movement 1

Turn your body slightly to the right, to the 10 o'clock position. Draw your right hand back in a curve in front of your chest with the palm turned down. Turn your left palm up and bring it across your waist in a curve to "hold a ball," with your right hand on top. At the same time, bring your left foot a half step toward your right foot.

Movement 2

Bring your left heel down and gently lean your upper body back, shifting your weight onto your left leg (middle photo). Turn your body slightly to the left, to 8 o'clock, and move your right foot slightly forward, resting your toes lightly on the floor to form a right empty step. Both legs should be bent slightly at the knees.

Movement 3

As you turn your body slightly back to the right, to 9 o'clock, slowly raise your left hand in front of you, toward your left temple, with the palm turning outward (bottom photo). Move your

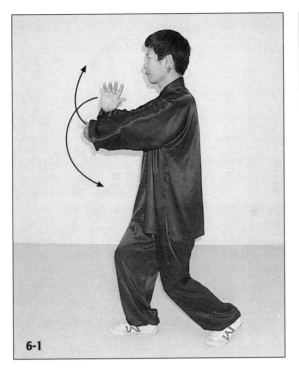

6-1

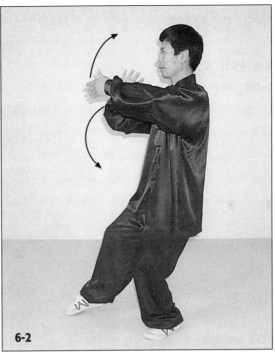

6-2

right hand down to your right hip with your palm turning down and your fingers pointing forward. Look to the front.

✔ Key Points

1. Do not thrust your chest forward or raise your shoulders. Keep your elbows down.

2. As you shift your weight forward, this should be coordinated with placing your arms in the hold-ball position. As you shift your weight backward, you should simultaneously lower the right palm and raise your left palm.

3. Round your arms when separating your hands. Prop up your left forearm and palm with flexible strength.

4. Face 9 o'clock in the final position.

✔ Self-Defense Application

Use your left hand and forearm to protect your head, chest, and upper left side from your attacker's punch. Use your right hand to block your abdomen and right hip, in case your attacker tries to kick your lower body. The motion is generated from the waist, not just the arms. The left arm moving up and spreading has the pur-

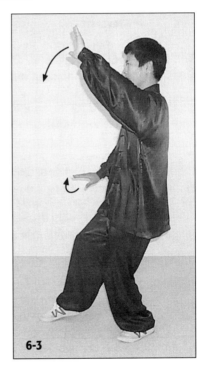

6-3

pose of warding off a blow. In coordination with the arm motion, you can also kick your attacker's lower body with your right foot, since all your body weight is on your left leg.

45

Posture 7

BRUSH KNEE
—RIGHT

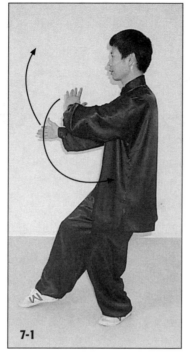

7-1

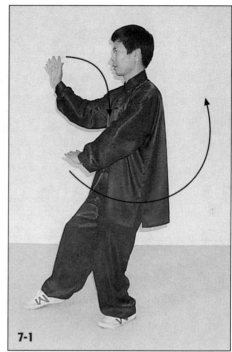

7-1

Movement 1

As your left hand moves in a curve to the right of your chest and then downward, turn your body slightly to the right, to 10 o'clock to lead the movement. Turn your body back to the left side, to 8 o'clock, to bring your right hand up in a curve to your left chest. While your body turns left, your left hand should circle past your abdomen, then up to ear level, with the arm bending slightly and the palm facing obliquely upward. Your right hand should continue its circle in a left-downward curve to the left side of your body, with the palm facing obliquely downward. Bring your right foot back, toes touching the floor.

Movement 2

Turn your body to the right to 9 o'clock as you step your right foot to the 10 o'clock position to form a right bow stance. Shift your major weight onto your right leg. At the same time, curve your left forearm and push your left hand forward by

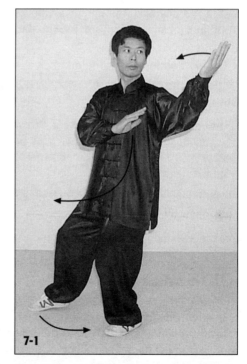

7-1

the side of your left ear at nose level, with the palm facing forward. Bring your right hand down in a circular motion and brush past your right knee, coming to rest beside your right hip. Look at the fingertips of your left hand.

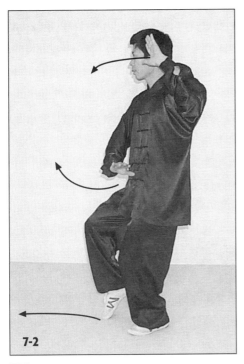

7-2

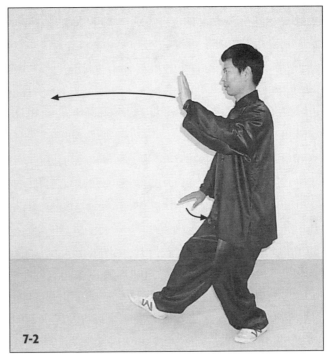

7-2

☑ Key Points

1. When your right foot steps out, push your left hand out as your body weight shifts forward. The left hand pushing depends more on the body movement than on the arm.

2. Keep a transverse distance of 12 inches between your heels in a bow stance to hold a firm balance and an easy energy flow.

3. Keep your body erect. Drop your shoulder and keep your elbows down. Relax your waist and hips.

4. The left arm moves in a clockwise circle and the right arm moves in a counter-clockwise circle. Remember, your body's turn initiates your arm's motion.

5. Face 9 o'clock in the final position.

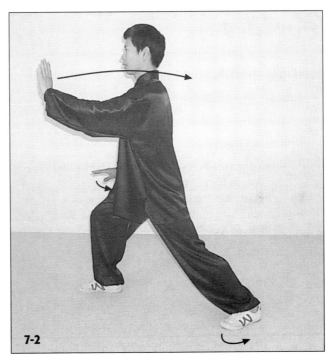

7-2

☑ Self-Defense Application

Block your attacker's punches by using your left arm, moving down and to the right, and your right arm, moving up and to the left. Both blocks are energized by your waist, not your arms. Following the two blocks, step your right foot forward to push your attacker with your left palm.

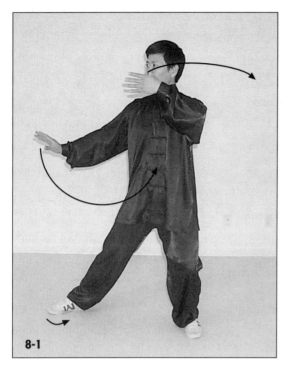

8-1

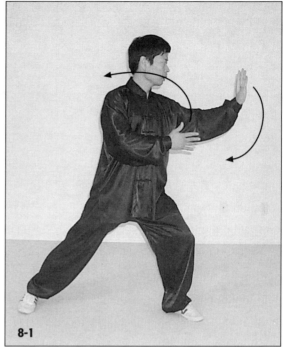

8-1

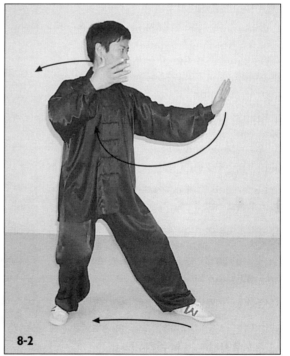

8-2

Posture 8

SINGLE WHIP

Movement 1

Rotate your left toes outward slightly as you sit back and shift your body weight gradually onto your left leg. Turn your right toes inward. Turn your body to the left, to 5 o'clock, and move your left hand back.

Move both hands to the left, with your left hand on top and your right hand at abdomen level, until your left arm is extended sideways at shoulder level, with the palm turning outward. Bend your right arm at the elbow and curve your right hand up in front of your left ribs, with the palm facing obliquely inward and to the left. Look at your left hand.

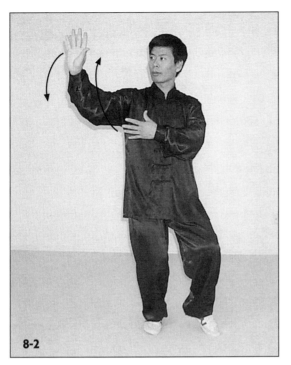

8-2

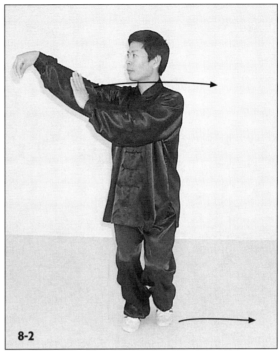

8-2

Movement 2

Shift your body weight slowly onto your right leg and turn your body to the right, to 7 o'clock. Bring your left foot back, next to your right foot, with its toes touching the ground. At the same time, move your right hand up in a curve to the upper side of your body.

    With palm turned outward, bunch your right fingertips and bend your wrist to form the hook of a bird beak. Move your left hand in a curve past your abdomen, up to the front of your right shoulder, with the palm facing inward.

Movement 3

Turn your body to the left, to 4 o'clock. Step out with your left foot toward 2 o'clock. Shift your body weight onto your left leg to form a left bow stance. Turn your right heel outward slightly to

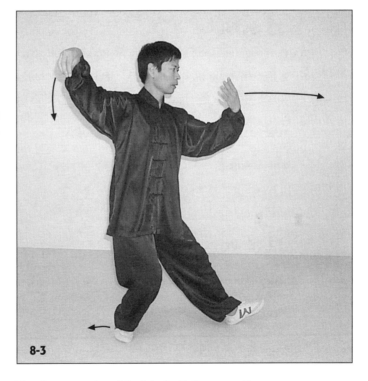

8-3

make sure your toes are pointing to a position between 4 and 5 o'clock. At the same time,

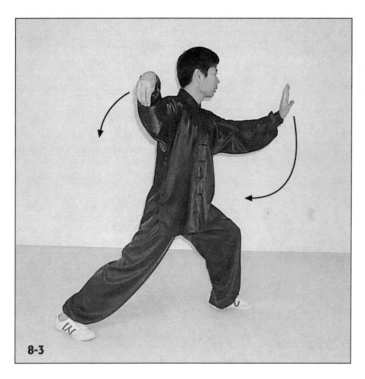

8-3

turn your left palm outward and push it out to the left, with its fingertips at eye level. Push and brace your right hooked hand toward 8 o'clock. Look at your left hand.

✔ Key Points

1. Mimic the motion of a whip. Swing your left arm out in coordination with turning your body.

2. Bend both arms slightly in the final position to keep your shoulders and elbows down. Your left elbow should be directly above your left knee.

3. As you push your left palm out, this should be synchronized with shifting your body weight forward to form the bow stance. The push is, therefore, powered by the body flow instead of the arm. Pushing energy comes from your feet, through your waist, and up to your left shoulder and arm.

4. Face 3 o'clock in the final position.

✔ Self-Defense Application

Move your arms in circles as your body and waist turn to block and intercept your attacker's hands. You can apply a splitting hit as you turn your palms outward. When stepping out and turning left, whip your left arm out like a strap to the left and then turn the palm to push and strike your attacker's neck area.

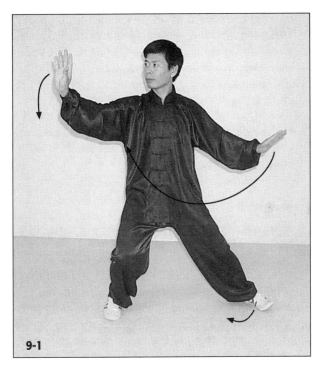

9-1

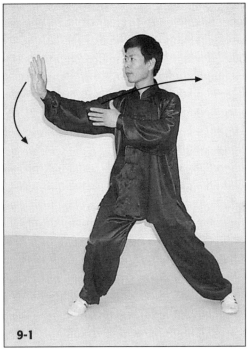

9-1

Posture 9

WAVE HANDS LIKE CLOUDS IN CIRCLE

9-2

Movement 1

Shift your body weight onto your right leg gradually, and turn your body to the right, to 7 o'clock. At the same time, turn your left toes inward and move your left hand in a downward curve past your abdomen and up to the front of your right shoulder, with your palm turning obliquely inward. Open your right hooked hand with the palm facing outward. Look at your right hand.

Movement 2

Turn your body gradually to the left, to 6 o'clock. Shift your weight onto your left leg.

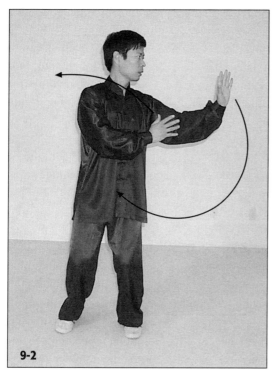

9-2

At the same time, move your left hand up and to the left in a curve, passing your face, with the palm turning out and to the left, while moving your right hand in a downward circle, passing your abdomen and then up to the front of your left shoulder, with the palm slowly turning inward. As your right hand circles upward, bring your right foot to the side of your left foot, so that they are parallel and about 10 inches apart. Both feet should face 6 o'clock. Look to the left.

Movement 3

Shift your weight onto your right leg and turn your body gradually to the right, to 7 o'clock. Move your right hand across your face in a curve, to the right side, with the palm turning slowly out and to the right. At the same time, move your left hand in a downward and upward curve across your abdomen, with the palm turning slowly inward.

As your left hand moves up, step your left foot back to 1 o'clock. Look at your left hand.

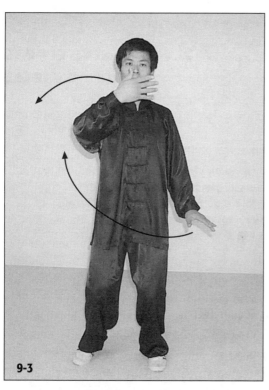

9-3

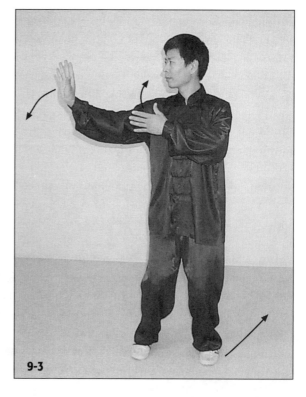

9-3

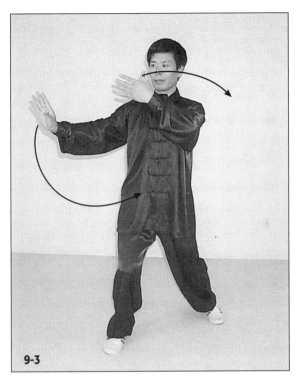

9-3

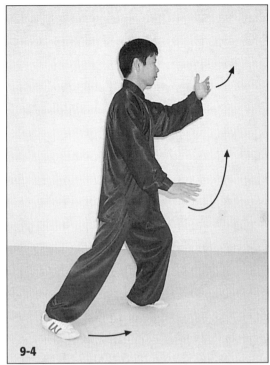

9-4

Movement 4

Turn your body to the left to 3 o'clock and shift your weight onto your left leg. At the same time, move your left hand up and to the left in a curve, passing your face, with the palm turning out and to the left, while moving your right hand in a downward circle, passing your abdomen and then up to the front of your left shoulder, with the palm slowly turning inward. As your right hand circles upward, bring your right foot to the side of your left foot, so that they are parallel and about 10 inches apart. Both feet should face 3 o'clock. Look to the left.

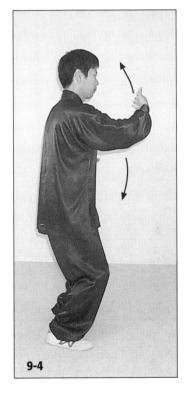

9-4

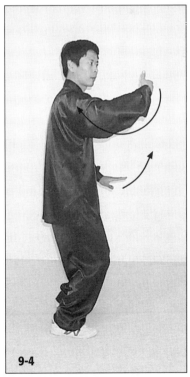

9-4

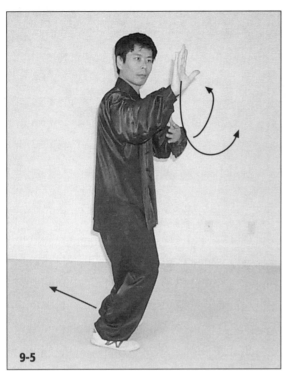

9-5

Movement 5

Shift your weight onto your right leg and turn your body gradually to the right, to 4 o'clock. Move your right hand across your face in a curve, to the right side, with the palm turning slowly out and to the right. At the same time, move your left hand in a downward and upward curve across your abdomen, with the palm turning slowly inward.

Movement 6

As your left hand moves up, step your left foot back to 10 o'clock. Look at your left hand.

Movement 7

Turn your body gradually to the left, to 12 o'clock. Shift your weight onto your left leg.

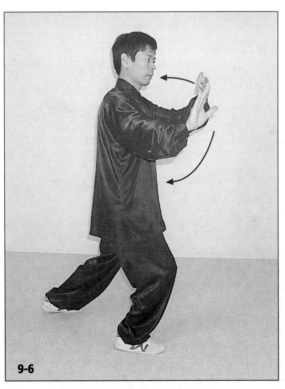

9-6

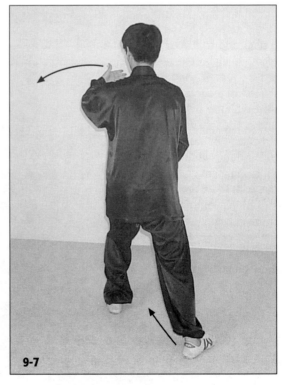

9-7

Movement 8

Move your left hand up and to the left in a curve, passing your face, with the palm turning out and to the left, while moving your right hand in a downward circle, passing your abdomen and then up to the front of your left shoulder, with the palm slowly turning inward. As your right hand circles upward, bring your right foot to the side of your left foot, so that they are parallel and about 10 inches apart. Both feet should face 12 o'clock. Look to the left.

Movement 9

Shift your weight onto your right leg and turn your body gradually to the right, to 1 o'clock. Move your right hand across your face in a curve, to the right side, with the palm turning slowly out and to the right. At the same time, move your left hand in a downward and upward curve across your abdomen, with the palm turning slowly inward.

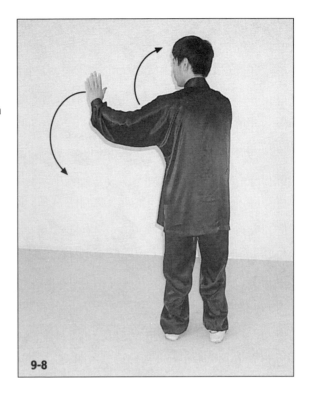

9-8

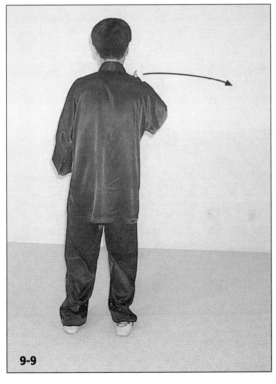

9-9

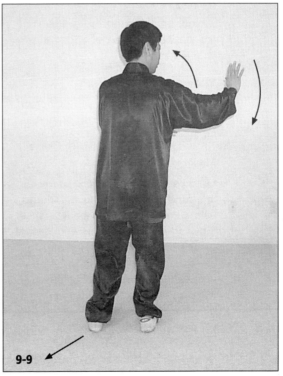

9-9

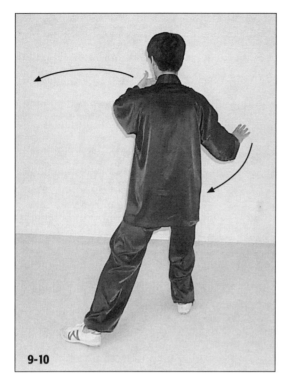

9-10

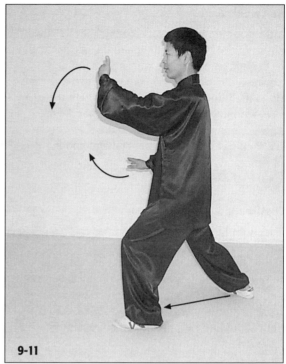

9-11

Movement 10

As your left hand moves up, step your left foot back to 7 o'clock. Look at your left hand.

Movement 11

Turn your body gradually to the left, to 9 o'clock. Shift your weight onto your left leg.

Movement 12

Move your left hand up and to the left in a curve, passing your face, with the palm turning out and to the left, while moving your right hand in a downward circle, passing your abdomen and then up to the front of your left shoulder, with the palm slowly turning inward. As your right hand circles upward, bring your right foot to the side of your left foot, so that they are parallel and about 10 inches apart. Both feet should face 9 o'clock. Look to the left.

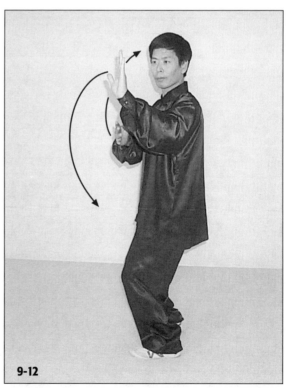

9-12

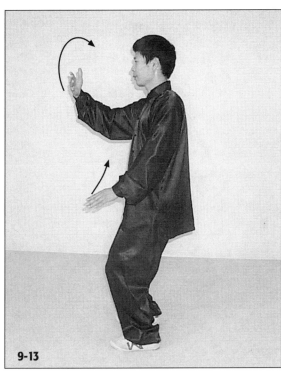

9-13

Movement 13

Shift your weight onto your right leg and turn your body gradually to the right, to 10 o'clock. Move your right hand across your face in a curve, to the right side, with the palm turning slowly out and to the right. At the same time, move your left hand in a downward and upward curve across your abdomen, with the palm turning slowly inward.

Movement 14

As your left hand moves up, step your left foot back to 4 o'clock. Look at your left hand.

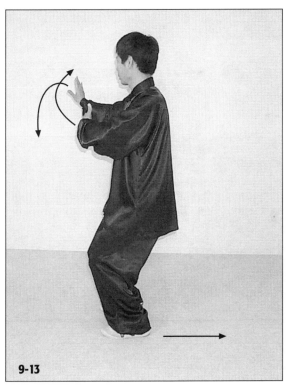

9-13

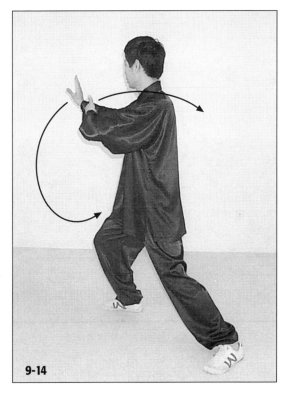

9-14

Movement 15

Turn your body gradually to the left, to 6 o'clock. Shift your weight onto your left leg.

Movement 16

Move your left hand up and to the left in a curve, passing your face, with the palm turning out and to the left, while moving your right hand in a downward circle, passing your abdomen and then up to the front of your left shoulder, with the palm slowly turning inward. As your right hand circles upward, bring your right foot to the side of your left foot, so that they are parallel and about 10 inches apart. Both feet should face 6 o'clock. Look to the left.

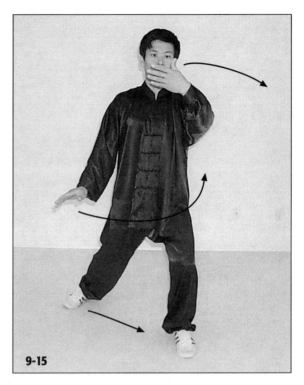

9-15

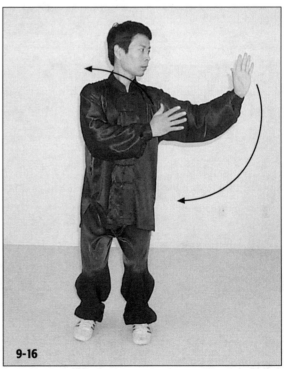

9-16

☑ Key Points

1. The nine major joints in your body (waist, spine, neck, hips, knees, ankles, shoulders, elbows, and wrists) turn together at the same slow pace. Keep your waist and hips relaxed and your shoulders down.

2. Initiate the waving-hands motion with your waist and use your lumbar spine as the axis on which your body turns. Your arms and hands should move as your waist turns. Keep both arms in a round and natural position. Each hand draws a circle, overlapping in front of your body.

3. Keep your body weight on your right leg when stepping your left foot to the back corner. Keep your body weight on your left leg when bringing your right foot in. Maintain a good balance when you make the steps.

4. The steps form a square and turn, in a counterclockwise motion, through four points: from the initial 6 o'clock position, to 3 o'clock, to 12 o'clock, to 9 o'clock, then back to 6 o'clock. This is different from the classic Tai Chi forms, which require a lot of space due to stepping side-to-side and facing only two directions. This square format compresses the classic Tai Chi form and requires much less practice space.

5. Your eyes should follow whichever hand is moving across your face.

6. Face 6 o'clock in the final position.

☑ Self-Defense Application

First, move your arms in a circle to block and protect your front body—from your lower abdomen to your upper chest and face. Second, turn your arms outward to apply the pushing and splitting force when your hand passes your face. Remember, keep your shoulder, elbow, and wrist in a relaxed condition for an easy and fast energy flow to your palm. Your waist and spine energize the pushing and splitting. This provides more power for throwing your attacker off balance. Waving your hands in a circle allows you to fight more than one attacker coming from different directions.

Posture 10

GRASP BIRD'S TAIL—LEFT

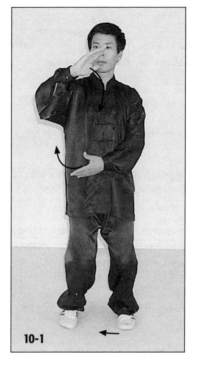

10-1

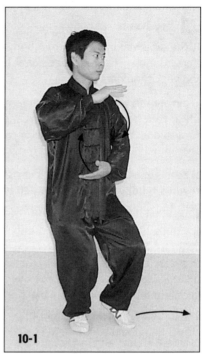

10-1

Movement 1

Shift your body weight onto your right leg and turn your body slightly to the right, to 7 o'clock. At the same time, move your right hand upward in a curve, across your face to your shoulder on the right side. Turn your right hand around, with the palm facing down. At the same time, move your left hand down in a curve, past your abdomen, while turning the palm up to form a hold-ball posture with your right hand, in front of the right side of your chest. Draw your left foot to the side of your right foot, with its toes on the floor. Look at your right hand.

Movement 2

Turn your body slightly to the left and step your left foot to 2 o'clock. Continue turning your body to the left, to 3 o'clock, and shift your weight onto your left leg to form a left bow stance. Move your left forearm up to shoulder level, with your palm facing inward and your elbow bending as if warding off a coming attack, while dropping your right hand slowly to the side of your right hip, with the palm facing down. Look at your left forearm.

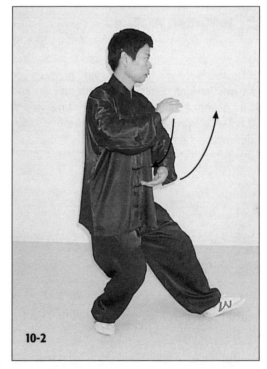

10-2

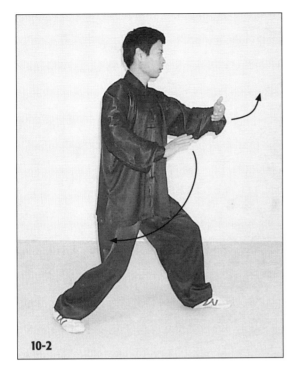

10-2

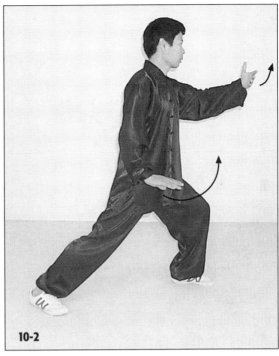

10-2

✓ Key Points

1. Make sure your left heel touches the floor first when taking the left step. As your body weight shifts forward, press down your left sole to make your whole left foot touch the floor.

2. Keep both arms rounded. Keep your shoulders and elbows sunk.

3. Coordinate your hands' separation with your body's turning and your left leg's bending.

4. Keep a 12-inch transverse distance between your feet when forming the bow stance.

5. Face 3 o'clock in the final position.

✓ Self-Defense Application

This is called the "Ward Off" movement. Use your left forearm to intercept your attacker's hand and dissolve the force by turning your body to the left. Bring your right arm down and lower your hand to protect yourself from your attacker's kick.

Grasp the Bird's Tail is composed of four techniques: ward off, roll back, press, and push. They are linked together to deflect an attack, and to pull or push an attacker off balance.

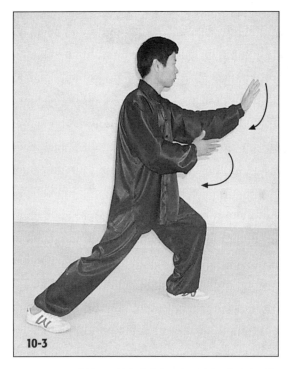

10-3

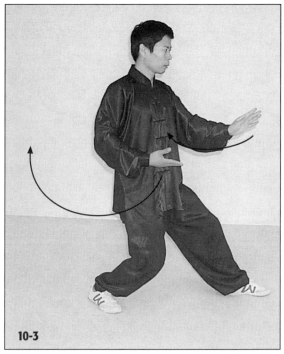

10-3

10-3

Movement 3

Turn your body slightly to the left, to a position between 2 and 3 o'clock, and extend your left hand forward, with the palm turning down as if grabbing something. Turn your right palm up and forward, and bring your right hand up across your abdomen until it is just below your left forearm. Then, turn your body slowly to the right, to 5 o'clock, and shift your weight back to your right leg. At the same time, pull both hands back, down, up, and to the right, in a curve, until your right hand is at shoulder level with the palm facing up, and your left hand is in front of your chest with the palm facing inward. Your eyes should follow your right hand.

☑ Key Points

1. Pull back both arms in a circular movement as your body turns and your weight shifts back.

2. Keep your left foot flat on the floor. Do not lean your body forward or protrude your buttocks. Maintain your body in the center and root your feet into the ground to keep them solid and your body flexible.

3. Face 5 o'clock in the final position.

☑ Self-Defense Application

This is called a "Roll Back" movement. It allows you to hold your attacker's elbow and wrist to destroy balance. The pulling is energized through turning your waist and shifting your body weight backward.

Movement 4

Turn your body slowly to the left, to 3 o'clock. Bend your right arm and bring your right hand to the inside of your left wrist. Shift your body weight back to your left leg into a left bow stance while pressing both hands forward, with your left palm facing inward and your right palm facing outward. Look at your left wrist.

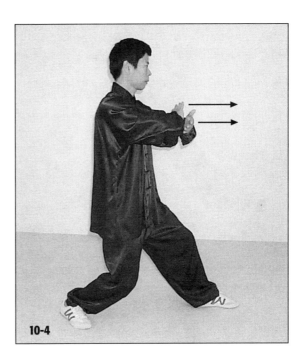

10-4

☑ Key Points

1. Pressing your hands forward must be coordinated with your body turning and your weight shifting forward. The pressing force comes from your waist and spine, in addition to your body weight. Press with a continuous pressure.

2. Keep both arms rounded and relaxed. Keep a 1-inch distance between your palms. Keep both shoulders sunk.

3. Keep your body erect. Do not lean forward when your hands press out. Keep both feet flat on the floor.

4. Face 3 o'clock in the final position.

☑ Self-Defense Application

This is called the "Press Out" movement. Use the flow of your body weight to press your left hand and forearm against your attacker's chest.

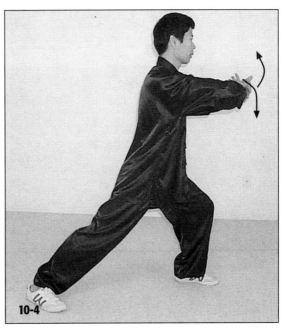

10-4

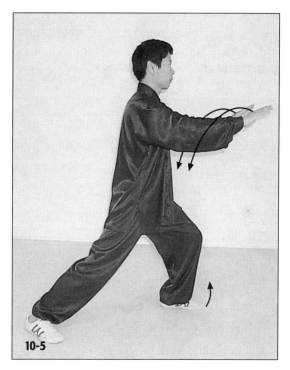

10-5

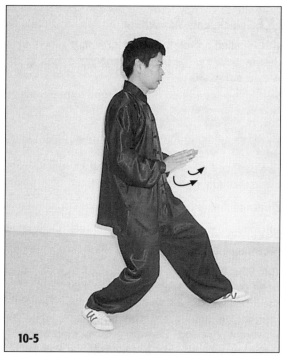

10-5

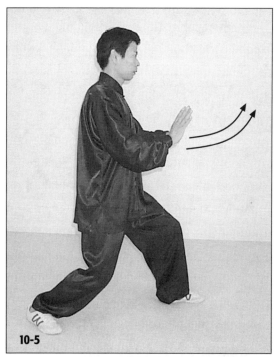

10-5

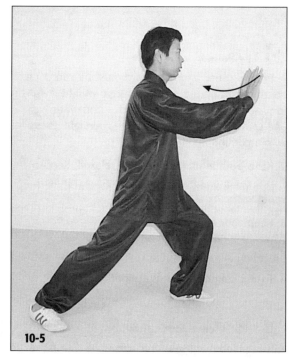

10-5

Movement 5

Following the press out motion, separate your hands to shoulder-width and turn both palms forward and down. Sit back and shift your weight onto your right leg, raising up your left toes. At the same time, draw both hands back and down in a curve to the front of your abdomen, with the palms pressing down. Transfer your body weight slowly onto your left leg, while pushing both palms forward and upward in a curve to shoulder level. Bend your left knee to form a left bow stance. Look to the front.

Key Points

1. Keep your waist and hips relaxed. Do not shrug your shoulder when pushing out your hands. Keep your elbows slightly down.

2. Coordinate your hands pushing with your body shifting forward. Use your body to generate the push instead of your arms.

3. Do not push your body weight too far forward. Your left knee should be behind your left toes.

4. Face 3 o'clock in the final position.

Self-Defense Application

This is called the "Push Out" movement. Sit back and draw your hands back to protect yourself and avoid an attack. Then, pin your attacker's arms down and push toward his chest. Push upward and forward to destroy the attacker's balance.

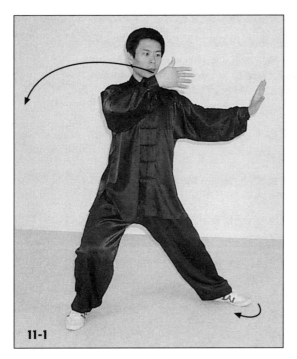

11-1

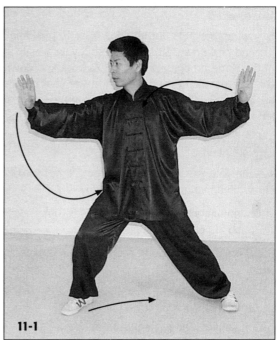

11-1

Posture 11

GRASP BIRD'S TAIL—RIGHT

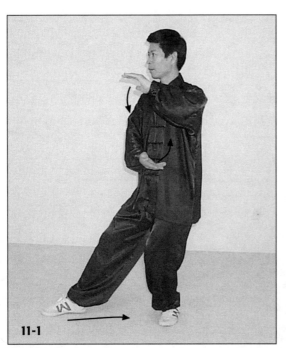

11-1

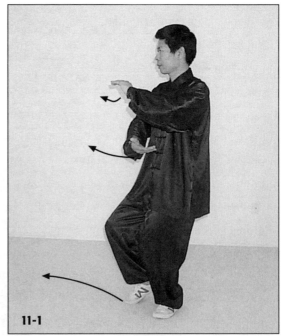

11-1

Movement 1

Sit back and turn your body to the right, to 6 o'clock. Shift your weight onto your right leg and turn your left toes inward. Move your right hand in a horizontal curve to the right, and then in a downward curve across your abdomen, turning your right palm up. Shift your weight back onto your left leg and bring your right foot next to your left, with its toes on the floor. Move your left hand inward, toward the right, to the front of your chest, and turn the palm down to form a hold-ball position with your right hand. Look at your left hand.

Movement 2

Turn your body slightly to the right and step your right foot to 10 o'clock. Continue turning your body to the right to 9 o'clock and shift your weight onto your right leg to form a right bow stance. Move your right forearm up to shoulder level, with your palm facing inward and your elbow bending as if warding off a coming attack, while dropping your left hand slowly to the side of your left hip, with the palm facing down. Look at your right forearm.

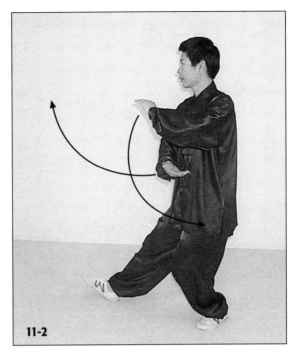

11-2

☑ Key Points

1. Make sure your right heel touches the floor first when taking the right step. As your body weight shifts forward, press down your right sole to make your whole right foot touch the floor.

2. Keep both arms rounded. Keep your shoulders and elbows sunk.

3. Coordinate your hands' separation with your body's turning and your right leg's bending.

4. Keep a 12-inch transverse distance between your feet when forming the bow stance.

5. Face 9 o'clock in the final position.

☑ Self-Defense Application

This is called the "Ward Off" movement. Use your right forearm to intercept your attacker's hand and

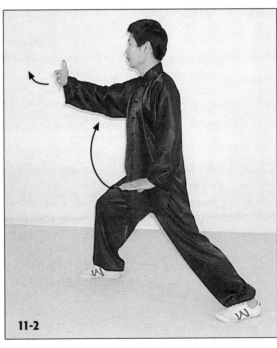

11-2

dissolve the force by turning your body to the right. Bring your left arm down and lower your hand to protect yourself from the attacker's kick.

Grasp the Bird's Tail is composed of four techniques: ward off, roll back, press, and push. They are linked together to deflect an attack, and to pull or push an attacker off balance.

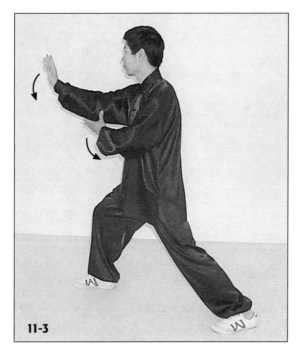

11-3

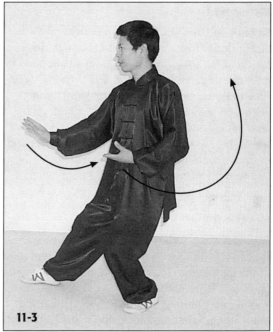

11-3

Movement 3

Turn your body slightly to the right , to a position between 9 and 10 o'clock, and extend your right hand forward, with the palm turning down, as if grabbing something. Turn your left palm up and forward, and bring your left hand up across your abdomen until it is just below your right forearm.

Then, turn your body slowly to the left, to 7 o'clock, and shift your weight back to your left leg. At the same time, pull both hands back, down, up, and to the left, in a curve, until your left hand is at shoulder level with the palm facing up, and your right hand is in front of your chest with the palm facing inward. Your eyes should follow your left hand.

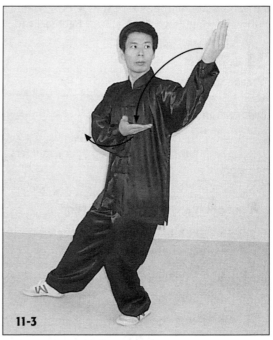

11-3

✓ Key Points

1. Pull back both arms in a circular movement as your body turns and your weight shifts back.

2. Keep your right foot flat on the floor. Do not lean your body forward or protrude your

buttocks. Maintain your body in the center and root your feet into the ground to keep them solid and your body flexible.

3. Face 7 o'clock in the final position.

☑ Self-Defense Application

This is called a "Roll Back" movement, which allows you to hold your attacker's elbow and wrist to destroy balance. The pulling is energized through turning your waist and shifting your body weight backward.

Movement 4

Turn your body slowly to the right, to 9 o'clock. Bend your left arm and bring your left hand to the inside of your right wrist. Shift your body weight back to your right leg into a right bow stance while pressing both hands forward with your right palm facing inward and your left palm facing outward. Look at the right wrist.

☑ Key Points

1. Pressing your hands forward must be coordinated with your body turning and your weight shifting forward. The pressing force comes from your waist and spine, in addition to your body weight. Press with a continuous pressure.

2. Keep both arms rounded and relaxed. Keep a 1-inch distance between your palms. Keep both shoulders sunk.

3. Keep your body erect. Do not lean forward when your hands press out. Keep both feet flat on the floor.

4. Face 9 o'clock in the final position.

☑ Self-Defense Application

This is called the "Press Out" movement. Use the flow of your body weight to press your right hand and forearm against your attacker's chest.

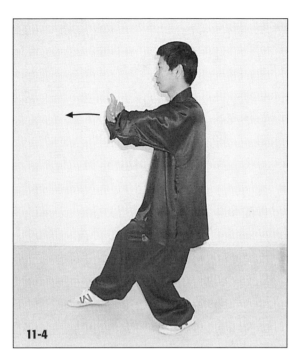

11-4

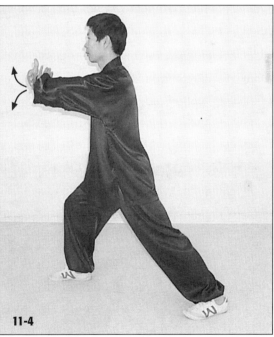

11-4

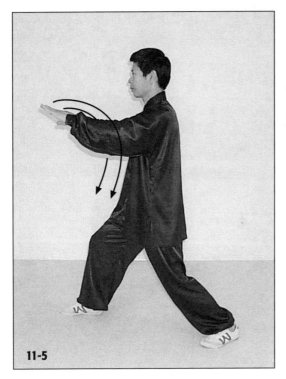

11-5

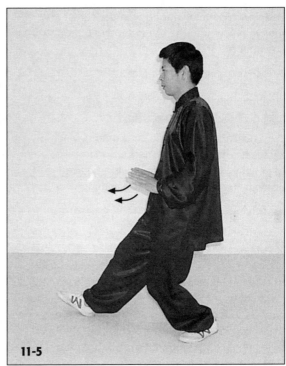

11-5

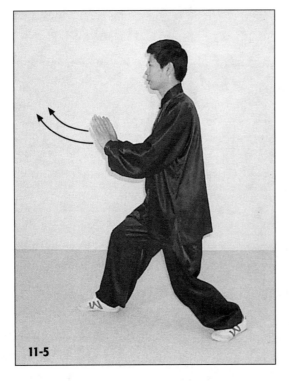

11-5

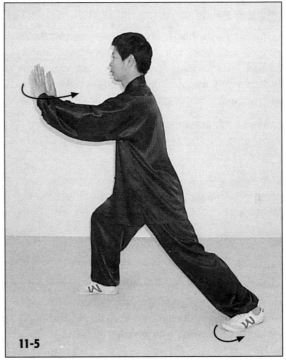

11-5

Movement 5

Following the press out motion, separate your hands to shoulder-width and turn both palms forward and down. Sit back and shift your weight onto your left leg, raising up your right toes. At the same time, draw both hands back and down in a curve to the front of your abdomen, with the palms pressing down. Transfer your body weight slowly onto your right leg, while pushing both palms forward and upward in a curve to shoulder level. Bend your right knee to form a right bow stance. Look to the front.

Key Points

1. Keep your waist and hips relaxed. Do not shrug your shoulder when pushing out your hands. Keep the elbows slightly down.

2. Coordinate your hands pushing with your body shifting forward. Use your body to generate the push instead of your arms.

3. Do not push your body weight too far forward. Your right knee should be behind your right toes.

4. Face 9 o'clock in the final position.

Self-Defense Application

This is called the "Push Out" movement. Sit back and draw your hands back to protect yourself and avoid an attack. Then, pin your attacker's arms down and push toward his chest. Push upward and forward to destroy the attacker's balance.

Posture 12

CROSS HANDS

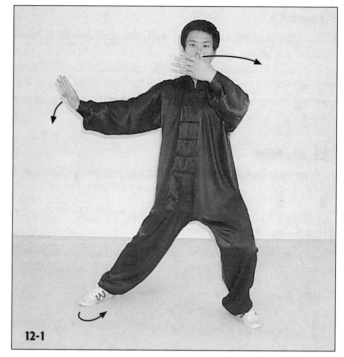

12-1

Movement 1

Rotate your left toes toward 6 o'clock, as you sit back and shift your body weight onto your left leg. Turn your body to the left, to 5 o'clock, with your right toes turning toward 6 o'clock. At the same time, move your left hand in a horizontal curve at shoulder level to your left side, with the left palm turning slowly outward and downward. Look at your left hand.

Movement 2

Shift your body weight slowly onto your right leg and bring your left foot toward your right foot, so they are parallel and a shoulder-width apart. Straighten both legs gradually and move both hands down

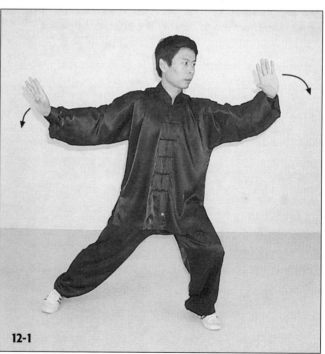

12-1

in a vertical curve to cross at the wrist in front of your abdomen. Then move your hands up to shoulder level with your right hand nearer your body, palms facing inward. Look to the front.

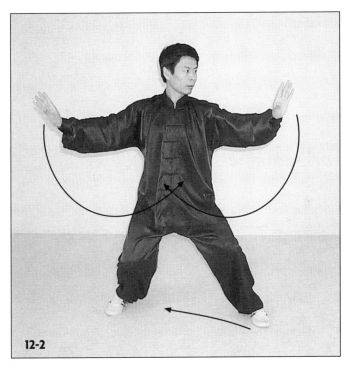

12-2

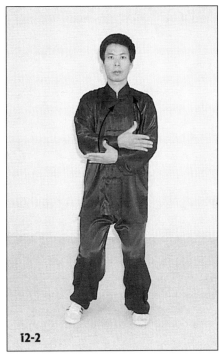

12-2

✅ Key Points

1. Place your weight evenly on both legs as your hands cross. Keep both arms in an arc shape, with elbows slightly bent.

2. Keep your body erect as you straighten your legs.

3. Face 6 o'clock in the final position.

✅ Self-defense Application

As you sit back and turn to the left, pull and grab your left hand to deflect an attack. Bring both hands down in a circular motion and then up to protect your front body.

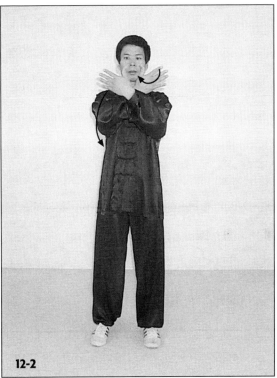

12-2

End of Sequence 1

It is optional to stop here, closing the form with Posture 74 (see page 226), or you can continue to practice with Sequence 2.

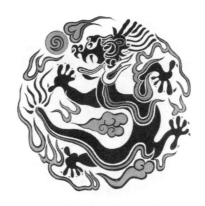

Sequence

2

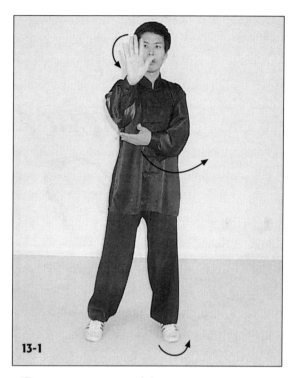

13-1

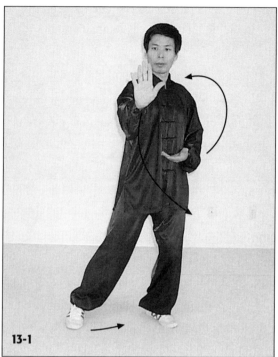

13-1

Posture 13

FAIR LADY WORKS WITH SHUTTLE—LEFT

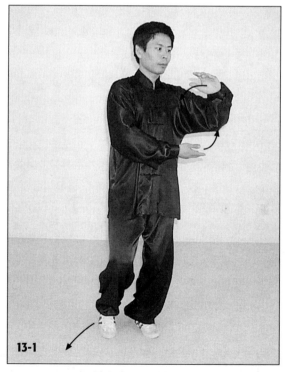

13-1

Movement 1

Shift your weight onto your right leg and rotate your left toes outward slightly. Then, shift your weight back to your left leg and bring your right foot next to your left, with its toes touching the floor. At the same time, rotate your right palm facing forward, while dropping your left hand down under your right elbow with the palm facing up. Turn your body to the left slightly, to 5 o'clock, and move both hands down in front of your body. Then move your left hand in an upward curve to the left, to the front of your left shoulder, with the palm facing down, while turning your right palm up to form a hold-ball position with your left hand. Look at your left forearm.

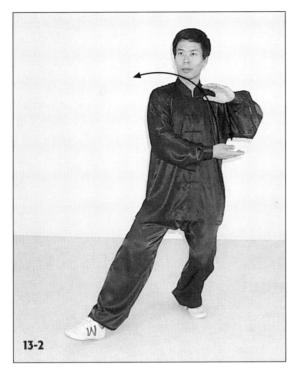

13-2

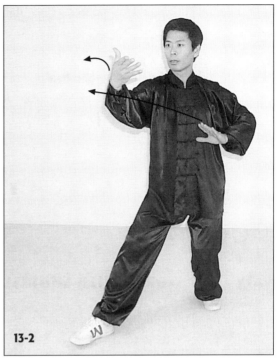

13-2

Movement 2

Turn your body slightly to the right and step your right foot toward 7 o'clock. Shift your weight slowly onto your right foot to form a right bow stance. At the same time, move your right hand up, crossing your face, to the right side of your forehead, with the palm rotating obliquely upward. Move your left palm in a small downward curve to the left before pushing it forward and up to nose level. Look at your left hand.

☑ Key Points

1. Coordinate your hand pushing with shifting your body weight forward and forming the bow stance.

2. Keep a transverse distance of about 12 inches between your heels in the bow stance for a good balance.

3. Don't lean your body forward while pushing out your hand. Don't raise your right shoulder when you raise your right hand to the side of your forehead.

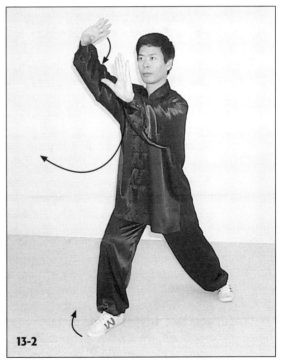

13-2

4. Push your left hand to 7 o'clock, the same direction in which your right toes are facing.

5. Face 7 o'clock in the final position.

☑ Self-Defense Application

Lift your right forearm to deflect your attacker's hand over your head. Step forward and strike your attacker's neck with your left palm. Remember to rotate your right hand while lifting it up. Make sure your right palm is facing upward and forward to form a strong protective arc.

Posture 14

FAIR LADY WORKS WITH SHUTTLE–RIGHT

Movement 1

Shift your body weight back onto your left leg. Turn your right toes slightly outward, to 8 o'clock. Shift your weight forward onto your right leg and bring your left foot next to your right, with its toes touching the floor. At the same time, move your left hand down and back in a curve to your right side at waist level to form a hold-ball position, with your right hand on top. Look at your right hand.

Movement 2

Turn your body slightly to the left and step your left foot toward 5 o'clock. Shift your weight slowly onto your left foot to form a left bow stance. At the same time, move your left hand up, crossing your face, to the left side of your forehead, with the palm rotating obliquely upward. Move your right palm in a small downward curve to the right before pushing it forward and up to nose level. Look at your right hand.

14-1

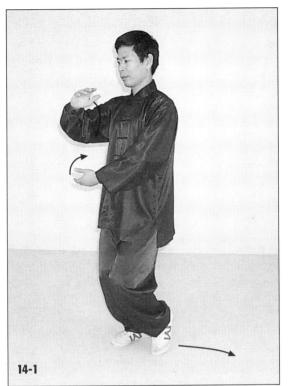

14-1

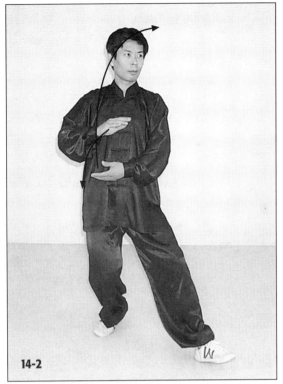

14-2

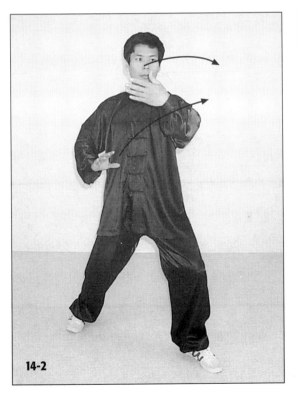

14-2

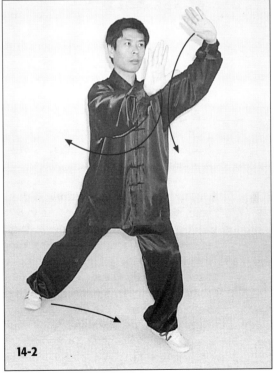

14-2

☑ Key Points

1. Coordinate your hand pushing with shifting your body weight forward and forming the bow stance.

2. Keep a transverse distance of about 12 inches between your heels in the bow stance for a good balance.

3. Don't lean your body forward while pushing out your hand. Don't raise your left shoulder when you raise your left hand to the side of your forehead.

4. Push your right hand to 5 o'clock, the same direction in which your left toes are facing.

5. Face 5 o'clock in the final position.

☑ Self-Defense Application

Lift your left forearm to deflect your attacker's hand over your head. Step forward and strike your attacker's neck with your right palm. Remember to rotate your left hand while lifting it up. Make sure your left palm is facing upward and forward to form a strong protective arc.

Posture 15

NEEDLE AT SEA BOTTOM

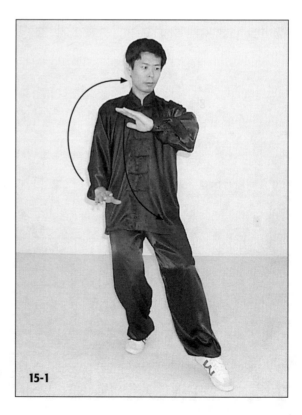

15-1

Bring your right foot a half step forward and shift your weight back onto your right leg. At the same time, adjust your left foot forward slightly, with its toes touching the floor to form a left empty stance. When you do so, turn your body slightly to the right, to 8 o'clock, with your left hand moving down and to the right, and your right hand moving down and back. Then, turn your body back to the left, to 6 o'clock. Move your left hand to the side of your left hip. At the same time, move your right palm in an upward curve from the right side to ear level, then drop it down in front of your body, fingers pointing down. Look at your right hand.

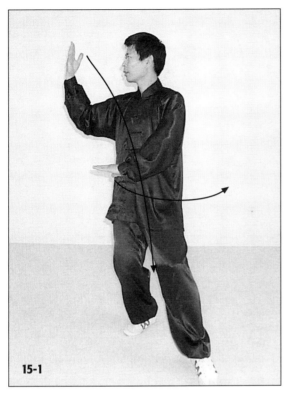

15-1

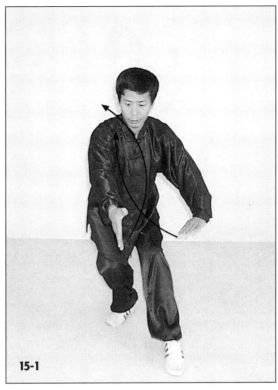

15-1

☑ Key Points

1. In the final position, do not lean your body too far. Keep your head erect.

2. Keep your weight on your back leg. Bend both knees as far as is comfortable.

3. Face 6 o'clock in the final position.

☑ Self-Defense Application

When an attacker punches you with his or her right hand, you block and grab that hand with your left hand and spear the attacker's low body with your right hand. If you are attacked with the left hand, you can intercept and grab the attacker's wrist with your left hand and then place your right forearm against that person's left elbow.

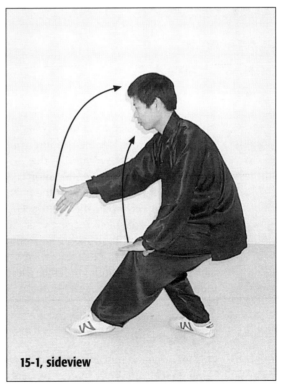

15-1, sideview

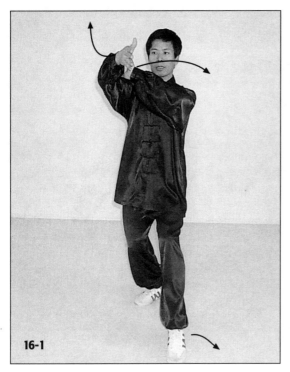

16-1

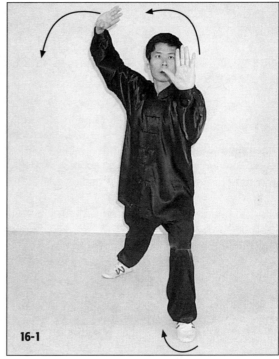

16-1

Posture 16

FLASH ARMS

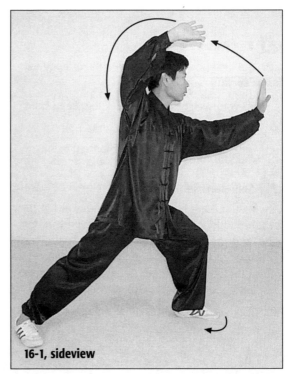

16-1, sideview

Turn your body slightly to the right and step your left foot forward to form a left bow stance, facing 6 o'clock. At the same time, raise your right hand up in front of your right temple with the palm turning obliquely upward and fingers pointing forward, while moving your left hand up to chest level. Then turn your left palm outward to push it forward at nose level. Look at your left hand. The bottom photo shows the transition to Posture 17.

✔ Key Points

1. Your left hand pushing should be coordinated with your body weight shifting forward into a bow stance. Your body motion powers the pushing.

2. Both arms should be in an arc shape. Keep your elbows dropped. This posture is also called "Fan through Back," because your arms are extended in a position that resembles a Chinese hand fan. The power is generated and passed through your back to your arms.

3. Keep your upper body erect, with your waist and hips relaxed.

4. Face 6 o'clock in the final position.

✔ Self-Defense Application

Intercept and grab your attacker's wrist with your right hand and step forward to strike the chest area with your left palm. The motion should be as quick as a flash when you apply it as a defense.

Posture 17

TURN TO DEFLECT DOWN, PARRY AND PUNCH

Movement 1

Sit back and shift your weight onto your right leg. Turn your body to the right, to 9 o'clock, and turn your left toes inward. Continue to turn your body to the right, to 11 o'clock. Shift your weight back to your left leg and move your right hand in a downward curve to the right, with fingers clenched into a fist, to cross your abdomen

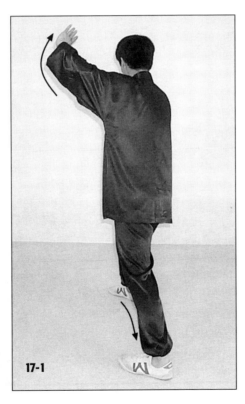 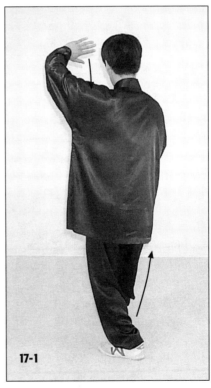

17-1   17-1

and move up to the left side of your ribs. At the same time, move your left hand up in a curve above your forehead, with the palm rotating obliquely forward. Look to the front.

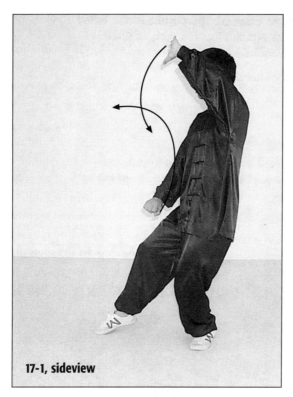

17-1, sideview

Movement 2

Lift your right foot and step it forward with its toes turning outward to 2 o'clock. Simultaneously, move your left hand down in front of your body, as if to deflect a punch. Then move it to the side of your left hip with the palm pressing down. Throw your right fist out in front of your chest for a back-hand punch toward 12 o'clock. Look at your right fist.

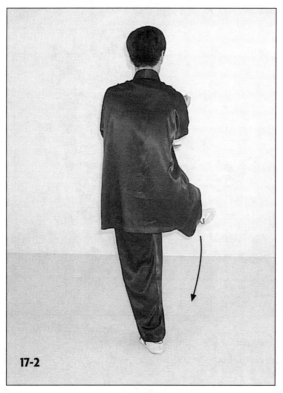

17-2

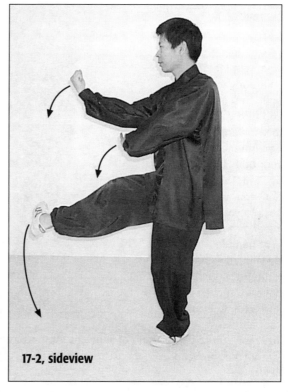

17-2, sideview

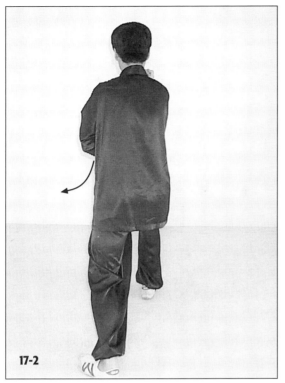

17-2

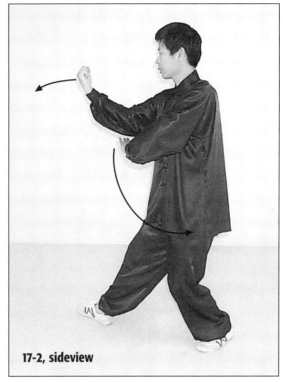

17-2, sideview

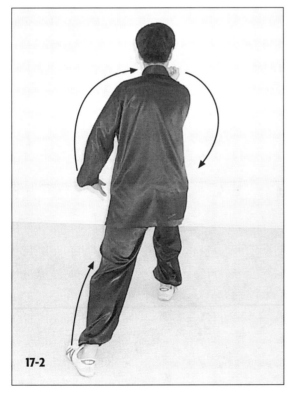

17-2

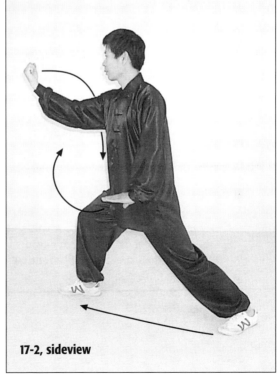

17-2, sideview

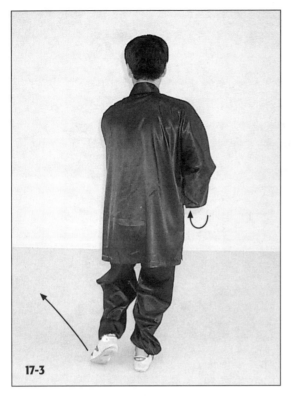

17-3

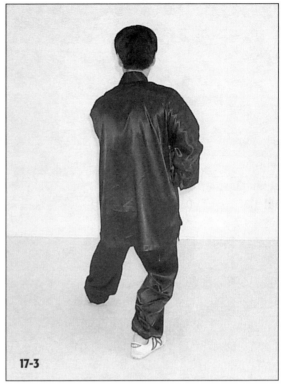

17-3

Movement 3

Shift your weight onto your right leg and step your left foot forward, to 11 o'clock. At the same time, move your left hand in an upward and forward curve to the right, to the front of your body, with the palm facing diagonally downward, while drawing your right fist back to the right side of your waist, its back facing downward. Look at your left hand.

Movement 4

Shift your weight forward onto your left leg to form a left bow stance as you strike your right fist forward at chest level with the fist eye facing upward. At the same time, pull back your left hand to the inside of your right forearm. Look at your right fist.

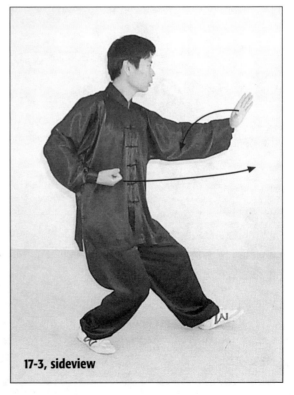

17-3, sideview

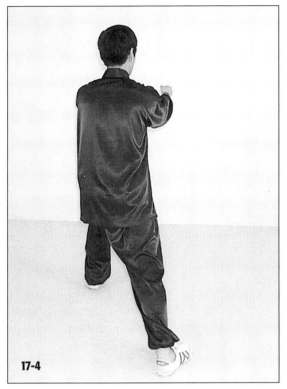

17-4

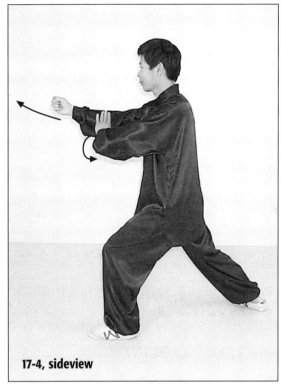

17-4, sideview

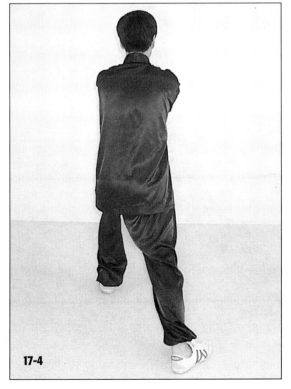

17-4

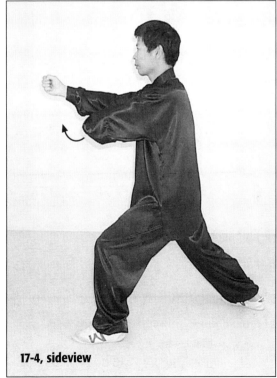

17-4, sideview

☑ Key Points

1. Striking out with your right fist should be coordinated with shifting your body weight forward. Power is emitted through your waist and back to your right fist.

2. Keep your shoulders and elbows relaxed. Do not straighten your right arm when you punch out with your right fist. Do not clench your fist too tightly.

3. Face 12 o'clock in the final position.

☑ Self-Defense Application

Turn 180 degrees to defend against an attacker approaching from the rear, using your left hand to deflect the arm downward. Follow up with a punch to the face with your right fist. At the same time, kick your attacker's knee with your right foot and step forward, intercepting the attacker's hand with your left hand and punching the chest with your right fist.

Posture 18

APPARENT CLOSING UP

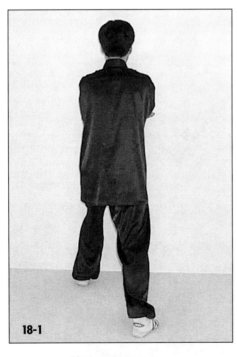

18-1

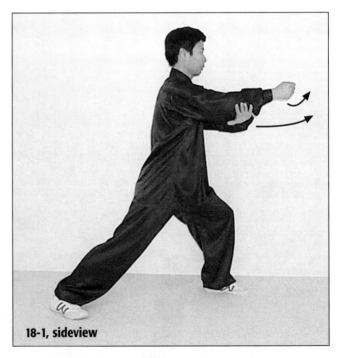

18-1, sideview

Movement 1

Slide your left hand down under your right elbow and turn your palm upward to stretch out

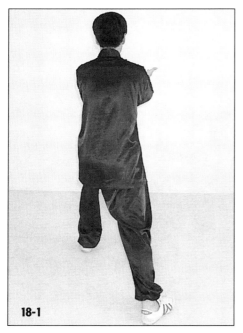

18-1

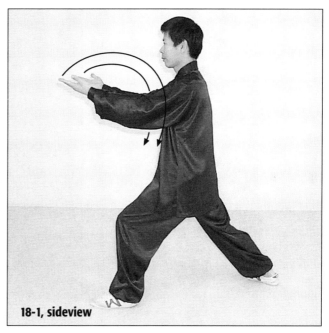

18-1, sideview

under your right forearm. At the same time, open your right fist and separate your hands about a shoulder-width.

Movement 2

Slowly withdraw both hands in a curve toward your chest. Sit back, shift your weight back onto your right leg, and raise your left toes. Draw your hands near your chest and turn the palms down, pressing down with both hands in front of your waist.

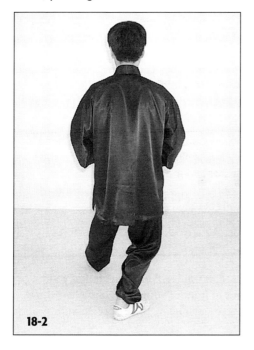

18-2

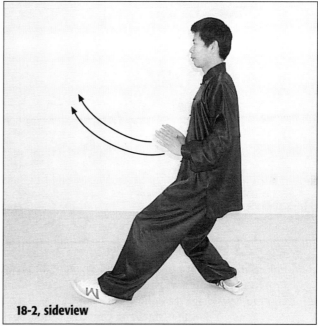

18-2, sideview

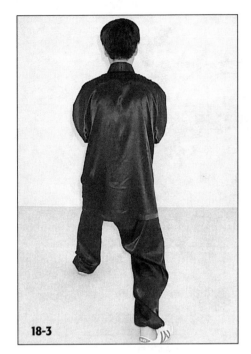

18-3

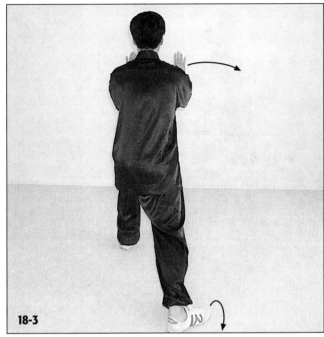

18-3

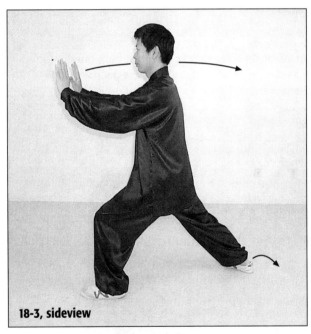

18-3, sideview

Movement 3

Shift your weight forward onto your left leg to form a left bow stance. Push both palms up and forward, until your wrists are at shoulder level. Look to the front.

☑ Key Points

1. Shifting your weight back to your right leg should be coordinated with drawing both palms toward your chest. Shifting your weight forward into a left bow stance should be coordinated with pushing both palms up and forward.

2. When you draw both hands back, bend your elbows slightly and keep them slightly away from your body.

3. Keep your upper body erect and hold your shoulders down.

4. Face 12 o'clock in the final position.

☑ Self-Defense Application

Slide your left hand down under your right elbow to protect yourself or to neutralize your attacker's hold on your right arm. Pull both hands back in front of your chest and press down to defend against an attacker's hands. Use both hands to push away in an upward and forward direction, throwing your assailant off balance.

Posture 19

BUMP WITH DIAGONAL LEAN TRUNK

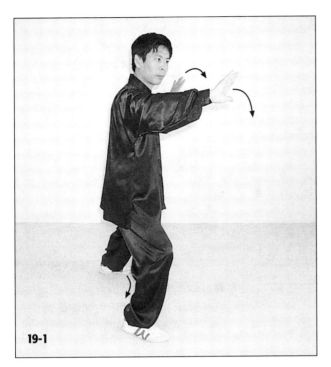

19-1

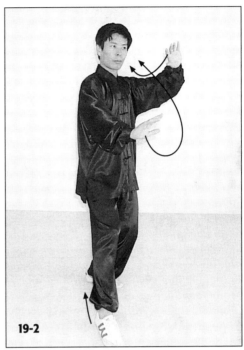

19-2

Movement 1

Rotate your right toes outward slightly as you turn your body to the right, to 3 o'clock, and shift your weight onto your right leg. Turn your left toes inward and move your right hand to the right in a curve with your palm rotating outward.

Movement 2

Shift your weight back to your left leg and bring your right foot next to your left, with its toes touching the floor. Move your right hand down and then move it up and to the left in a circular motion. Move your left hand in an upward curve to the right, then down in front of your chest, to cross your right hand. Both palms should be facing inward, with your right hand on the outside.

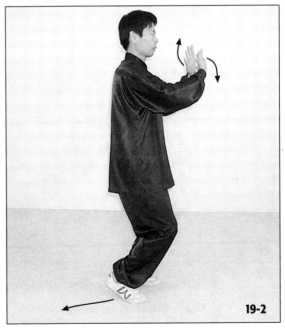

19-2

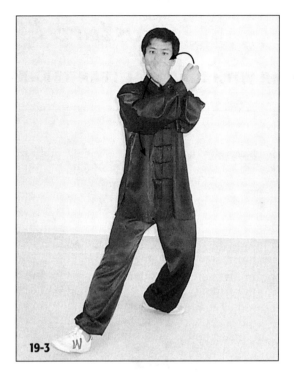

19-3

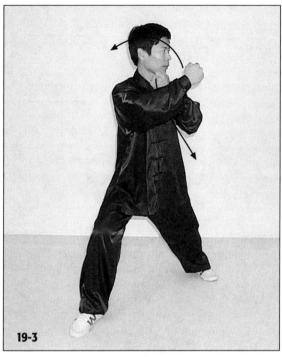

19-3

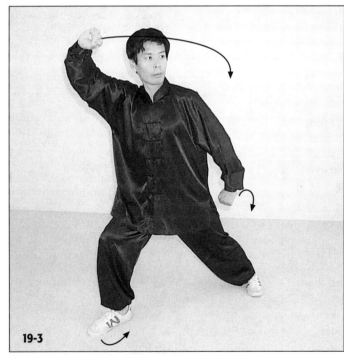

19-3

Movement 3

Turn your body to the right and step your right foot, toward 7 o'clock. Hold both hands in fists. Shift your weight to your right leg, assuming a right bow stance, while turning your body toward 5 o'clock. Strike out with your right shoulder. Extend your right fist up to your right temple, with the fist eye rotated downward. Lower your left fist to the side of your left hip. Look at your left side.

✅ Key Points

1. Do not lean too far forward with your upper body. Keep both feet rooted to the ground to hold a solid position.

2. Keep your shoulders sunk. Round both arms and maintain the supporting power.

3. The turning of your waist emits the bumping power. You can do it in a quick tempo.

4. Face 5 o'clock in the final position.

☑ Self-Defense Application

Move your right hand in a curve to your rear right quarter, while turning your body to the right to deflect an attack on your right side. Cross hands in front of your chest to protect your upper body. Step your right foot toward your attacker and strike with your right trunk and shoulder. At the same time, maintain both arms in an arc shape to protect yourself.

Posture 20

FIST UNDER ELBOW

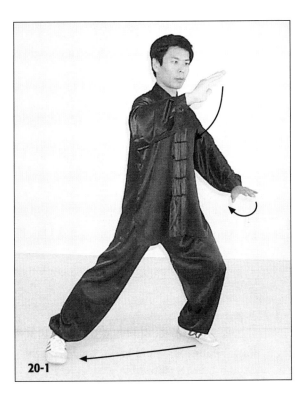

20-1

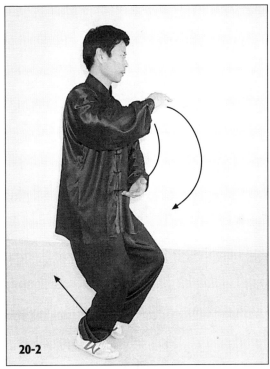

20-2

Movement 1

Shift your weight onto your left leg and turn your body back to the left, to 2 o'clock. At the same time, turn your right toes inward, drop your right elbow, and open both fists.

Movement 2

Shift your weight back onto your right leg, bringing your left foot next to your right, with its toes touching the floor. At the same time, bring both palms in front of your chest to form a hold-ball position. Look at your right hand.

93

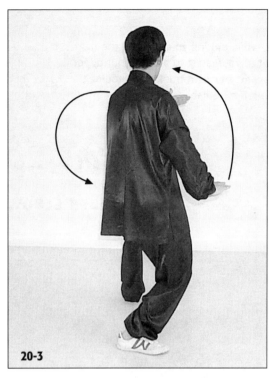

20-3

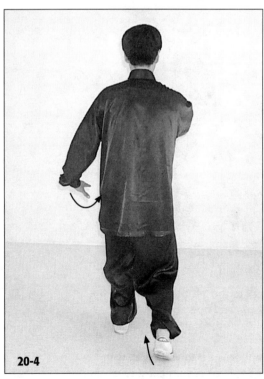

20-4

Movement 3

Step your left foot out to 11 o'clock, toes turned slightly outward, and turn your body to the left. Extend your left forearm up and forward in a curve, while lowering your right palm to your waist (arrows show transition to Movement 4).

Movement 4

Shift your body weight onto your left leg and move your right foot a half step forward, behind your left foot. At the same time, move your right palm up and forward, and pull your left palm back down to your waist.

Movement 5

Shift your weight back to your right leg and empty your left foot, its heel touching the floor. Extend your left palm up and forward and press down your right palm into a fist under your left elbow.

☑ Key Points

1. Shift your body weight back and forth twice in this transitional posture. Keep a good balance during the motion. Do not throw your buttocks out in the empty stance.

2. Keep your arms rounded and move them in coordination with your waist turning.

3. Your left palm should face your right at nose level in the final position.

4. Face 12 o'clock in the final position.

☑ Self-Defense Application

From the hold-ball position, step forward and ward off an attacker with your left forearm. Pull your right palm back and move it forward in a curve to intercept and press down an attacker's arm. Then, chop out your left forearm with the small finger facing forward.

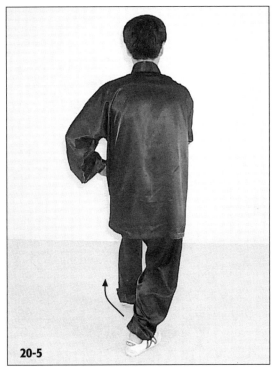

20-5

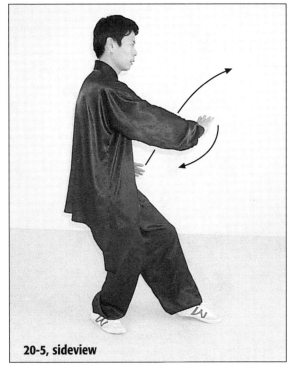

20-5, sideview

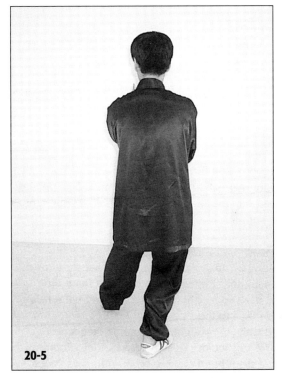

20-5

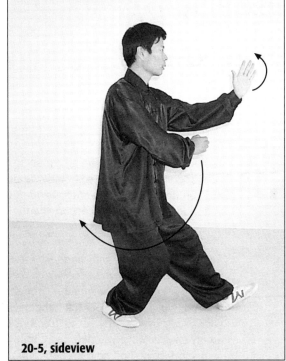

20-5, sideview

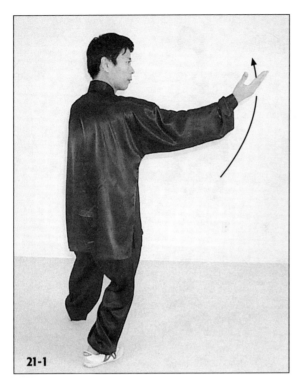
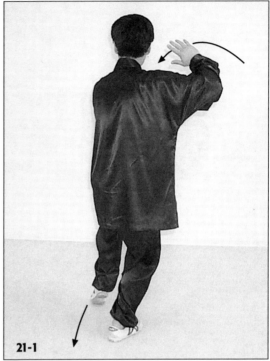

Posture 21

REPULSE MONKEY

Movement 1

Turn your body to the right, to 2 o'clock. Open your right fist and move it down in a curve past your abdomen, then up to shoulder level at your rear right. Rotate both palms to face up and hold up both arms with a slight bend at the elbows. Your eyes should first look to your right as your body turns in that direction, then at your left hand.

Movement 2

Raise your left foot slightly and take a step backward, to 7 o'clock. Place your left toes down first, then lower the whole foot slowly to the floor, toes turned outward. At the same time, bend your right arm toward your right ear and push your right hand out with the palm facing forward, while pulling your left hand back and down to the side of your left hip. Then, turn your body slightly to the left to 10 o'clock, and shift your weight onto your left leg for a right empty stance. Move your left hand up in a curve to shoulder level at your rear left. Rotate both palms to face up and hold up both arms with a slight bend at the elbows. Your eyes should first look to the left as your body turns in that direction, then at your right hand.

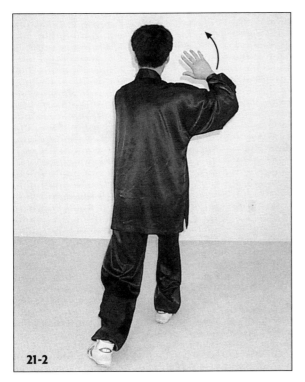

21-2

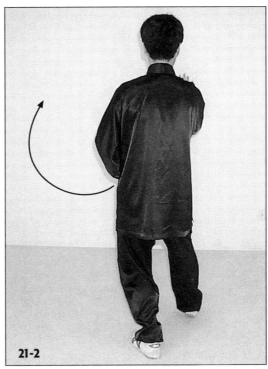

21-2

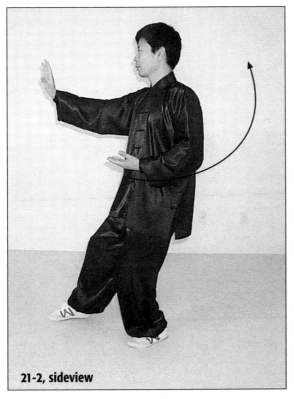

21-2, sideview

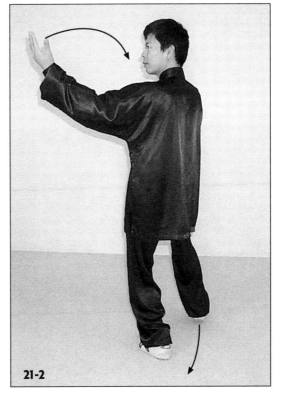

21-2

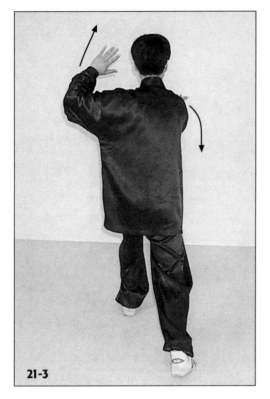

21-3

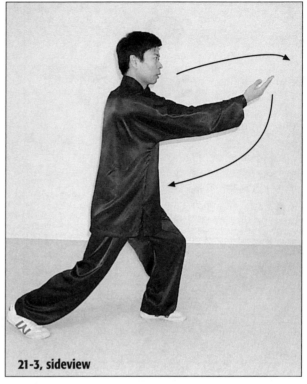

21-3, sideview

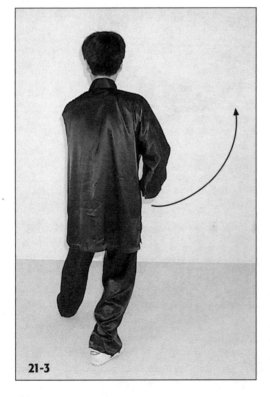

21-3

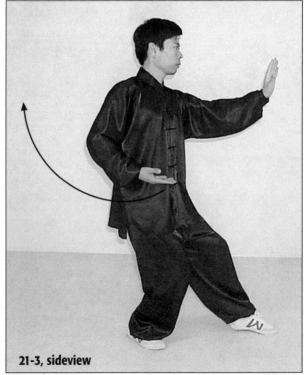

21-3, sideview

Movement 3

Raise your right foot slightly and take a step backward, to 5 o'clock. Place your right toes down first, then lower the whole foot slowly to the floor, toes turned outward. At the same time, bend your left arm toward your left ear and push your left hand out with the palm facing forward, while pulling your right hand back and down to the side of your right hip. Then, turn your body slightly to the right to 2 o'clock and shift your weight onto your right leg for a left empty stance. Move your right hand up in a curve to shoulder level at your rear right. Rotate both palms to face up and hold up both arms with a slight bend at the elbows. Your eyes should first look to the right as your body turns in that direction, then at your left hand.

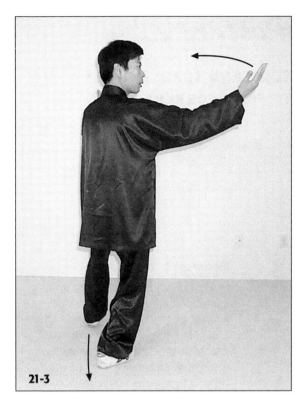

21-3

 Key Points

1. Keep your arms in a curve when pushing out or drawing back your palms. Do not lock your elbows.

2. When stepping back, place your toes down first, then gradually shift your weight back and make your whole foot touch the floor. When shifting your weight back, pivot on your front toes to make them point forward.

3. Keep your waist and hips relaxed. Move your foot a little sideways as you step back to prevent locking your hips.

4. Keep your eyes on the movement of your active hand. When your palms cross each other in front of your chest, try to sense the magnetic repulsion between them.

5. Face 12 o'clock in the final position.

 Self-Defense Applications

Use your front hand to intercept or grab an attacker's arm. Step back to pull an attacker over. Strike out with the other hand toward your attacker's head or chest.

Posture 22

TURN AND THRUST PALMS TO FOUR CORNERS

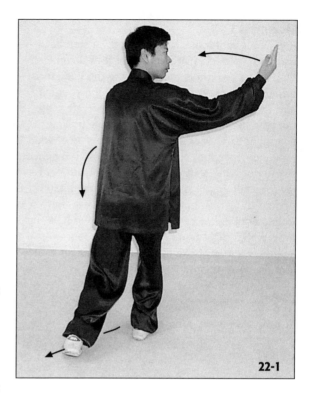

22-1

Movement 1

Move your left foot a half step back, to a position between 7 and 8 o'clock, with its toes touching the floor. At the same time, move your left palm back in an upward curve to the right, then down to the front of your right chest. Lift your right palm up to head level at your rear right.

22-2

Movement 2

Turn your body to the left, to 10 o'clock, by pivoting on your right heel and left toes. At the same time, bend your right palm toward your right ear and press your left hand down in front of your abdomen. Step your left foot forward, to a position between 7 and 8 o'clock, and shift your weight onto your left leg. Push your right palm out at shoulder level and move your left hand down and to the left, across the top of your left knee, bringing it to rest beside your left hip. Step your right foot a half step toward your left with toes touching the floor. Look at your right hand. Face a position between 7 and 8 o'clock.

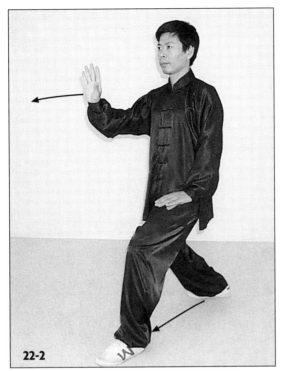

22-2

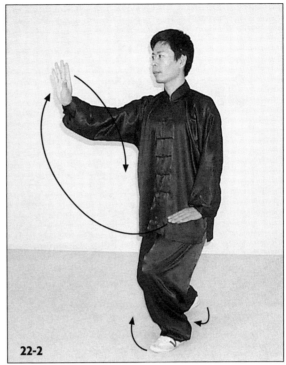

22-2

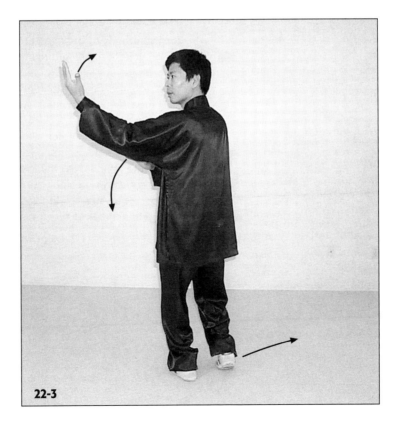

22-3

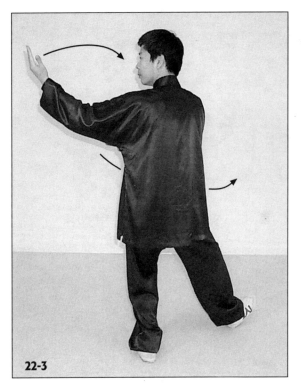

22-3

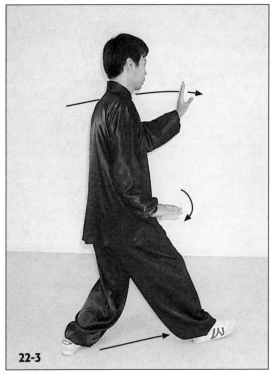

22-3

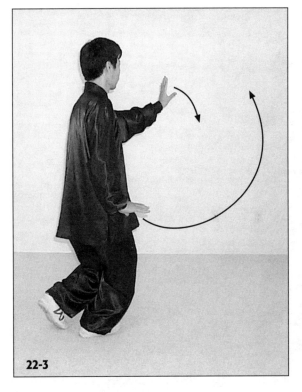

22-3

Movement 3

Turn your body to the right, to 11 o'clock, by pivoting on your left heel and right toes. At the same time, bend your left palm toward your left ear and press your right palm down in front of your abdomen. Step your right foot forward to a position between 1 and 2 o'clock and shift your weight onto your right leg. Push your left palm out at shoulder level and move your right hand down and to the right, across the top of your right knee, bringing it to rest beside your right hip. Step your left foot a half step toward your right, toes touching the floor. Look at your left hand.

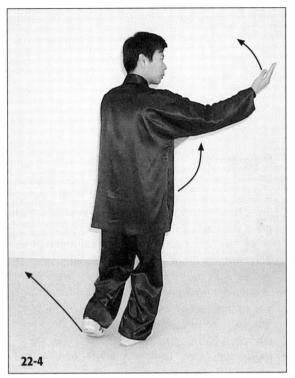

22-4

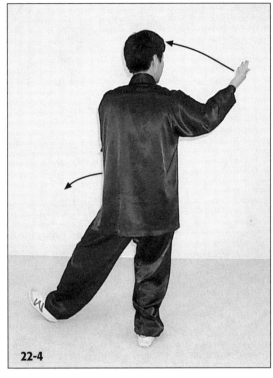

22-4

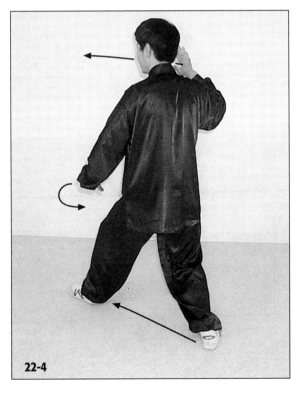

22-4

Movement 4

Move your right hand up from the rear right to shoulder level and turn your left hand toward your right chest. Then, step your left foot to a position between 10 and 11 o'clock and bend your right hand toward your right ear. Press your left hand down in front of your abdomen. Shift your weight onto your left leg and push your right hand out. At the same time, move your left hand down and to the left, across the top of your left knee, bringing it to rest beside your left hip. Then, step your right foot a half step toward your left, toes touching the floor. Look at your right hand. Face a position between 10 and 11 o'clock.

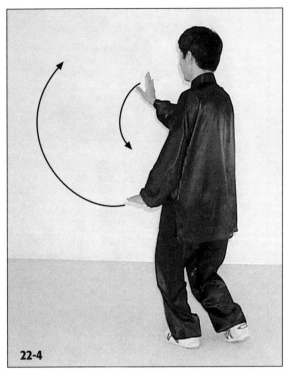

22-4

Movement 5

Turn your body to the right, to 2 o'clock, by pivoting on your left heel and right toes. At the same time, bend your left palm toward your left ear and press your right palm down in front of your abdomen. Step your right foot forward to a position between 4 and 5 o'clock and shift your weight onto your right leg. Push your left palm out at shoulder level and move your right hand down and to the right across the top of your right knee, bringing it to rest beside your right hip. Step your left foot a half step toward your right, with toes touching the floor. Look at your left hand.

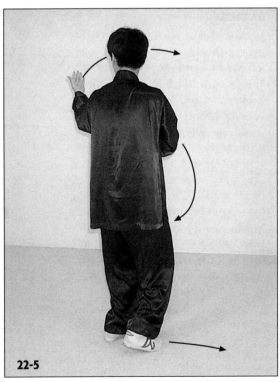

22-5

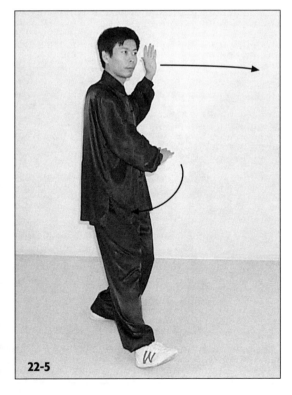

22-5

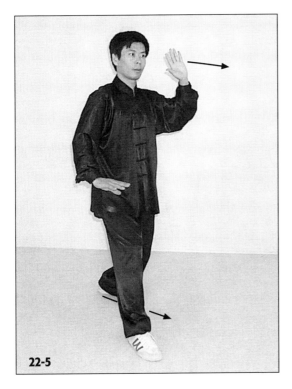

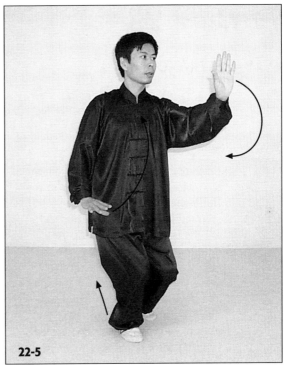

22-5

22-5

☑ Key Points

1. A major step followed by a half step is typical of the Sun Tai Chi style. It makes stepping more agile and smoother. This posture is called "Repulse Monkey," an old name from the Sun style.

2. When you take a half step forward, be sure to keep a 5-inch transverse distance between your feet in order to allow pivoting and turning.

3. When you push and thrust your palm, the movement should be coordinated with your body turning and your weight shifting forward.

4. Each push should move toward a diagonal corner. If you are facing south to start the form, your first push should be to the southwest, then the northeast, then the northwest, and finally the southeast.

5. Face a position between 4 and 5 o'clock in the final position.

☑ Self-Defense Application

Circle your front hand to block an attacker's punch, then step forward to thrust your other palm into the chest. Repeat the pushing into different corners in order to fight more than one attacker coming from different directions.

Posture 23

PLAY GUITAR–RIGHT

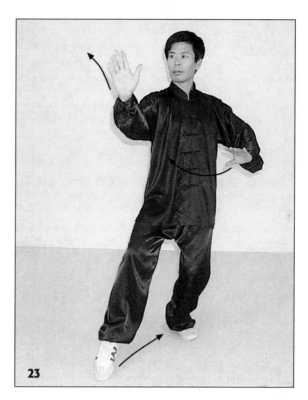

23

Turn your body slightly to the left and step back your left foot slightly in the same direction. Shift your weight onto your left leg and turn your body to the right, to 6 o'clock. Lift up your right foot and rest it on the heel to form a right empty stance. At the same time, move your left hand back in a downward curve and your right hand forward in an upward curve in front of your right chest, at nose level, with the palm facing left. Move your left hand up slightly toward your right elbow. Look at your right fingertips.

☑ Key Points

1. Hold your shoulders and elbows down. Coordinate your arms' motion with your waist turning.

2. Keep your body erect and natural, your chest relaxed. Bend both knees slightly in the empty stance.

3. Face 6 o'clock in the final position.

☑ Self-Defense Application

Intercept and grab an attacker's wrist using your left hand. Move your right palm up to hold and press the elbow against your left hand. Squeeze both palms in to bend the attacker's elbow.

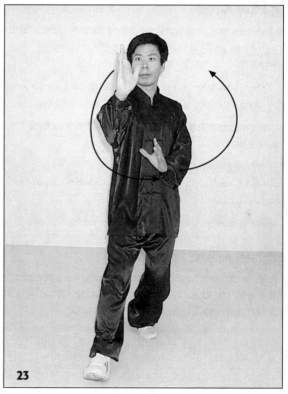

23

106

Posture 24

WHITE CRANE SPREADS ITS WINGS—LEFT

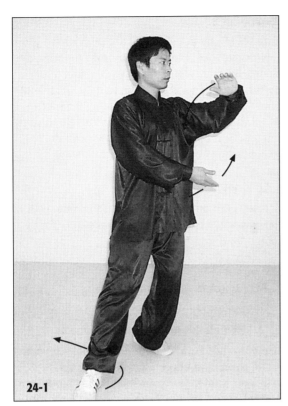

24-1

Movement 1

Turn your body slightly to the left, to 4 o'clock. Move your left hand down and to the left, then up in front of your chest in a circular motion, with the palm facing down. As you do so, move your right hand in a downward curve with the palm turning up to form a hold-ball position with your left hand. At the same time, bring your right foot back close to your left heel and take a half step toward 9 o'clock. Shift your weight onto your right leg and cross both forearms in front of your right chest. Look to the front.

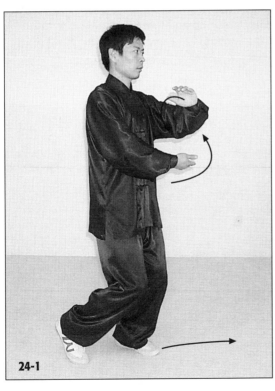

24-1

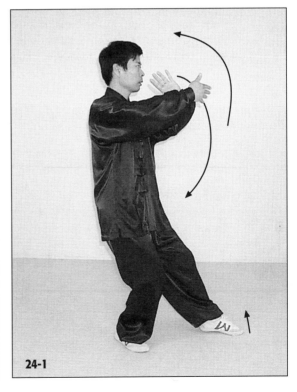

24-1

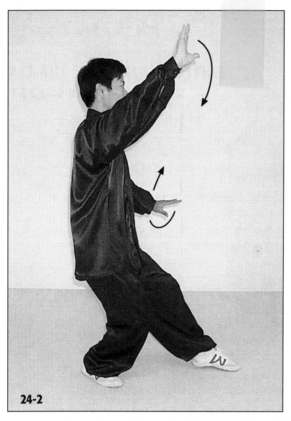

24-2

Movement 2

Turn your body to the left, to 3 o'clock. Move your left foot to your left side slightly, toes touching the floor, assuming a left empty stance. Move your right hand up and to the right, to the right side of your forehead, with the palm turning outward. Move your left hand down and to the left, to your left hip, with the palm turning down and the fingers pointing forward. Look straight ahead.

☑ Key Points

1. Keep both arms rounded and coordinate your arm movements with your body turning.

2. Do not thrust your chest forward or hold up your shoulders. Keep your elbows down.

3. Face 3 o'clock in the final position.

☑ Self-Defense Application

Use your right hand and forearm to protect your head, chest, and upper right side from your attacker's punch. Use your left hand to block your abdomen and left hip, in case your attacker tries to kick your lower body. The motion is generated from the waist, not just the arms. The right arm moving up and spreading has the purpose of warding off a blow. In coordination with the arm motion, you can also kick your attacker's lower body with your left foot, since all your body weight is on your right leg.

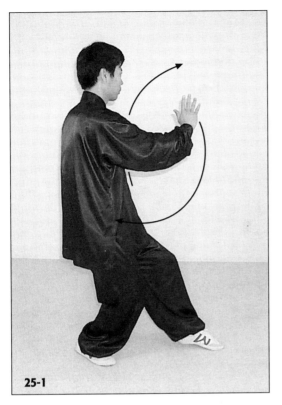

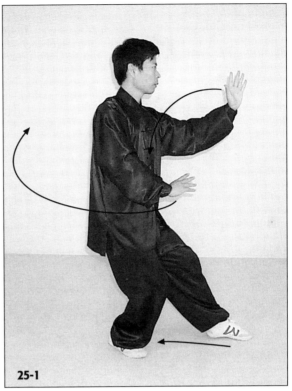

25-1

25-1

Posture 25

BRUSH KNEE–LEFT

Movement 1

As your right hand moves in a curve to the left of your chest and then downward, turn your body slightly to the left, to 2 o'clock, to lead the right hand movement. Turn your body back to the right side, to 4 o'clock, to bring your left hand up in a curve to your right chest. While your body turns right, your right hand should circle past your abdomen, then up to ear level, with the arm bending slightly and the palm facing obliquely upward. Your left hand should continue its circle in a right downward curve to the right side of your body, with the palm facing obliquely downward. Bring your left foot back, toes touching the floor.

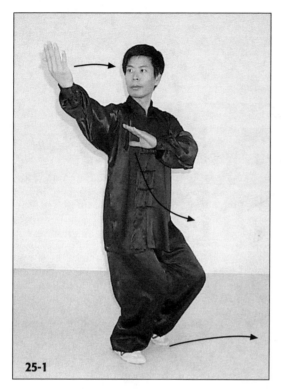

25-1

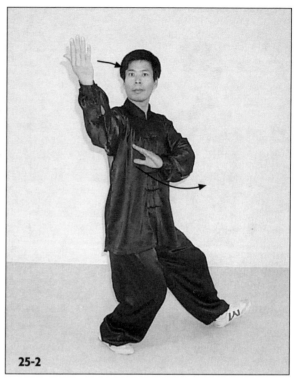

25-2

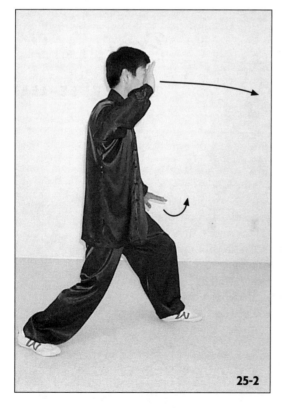

25-2

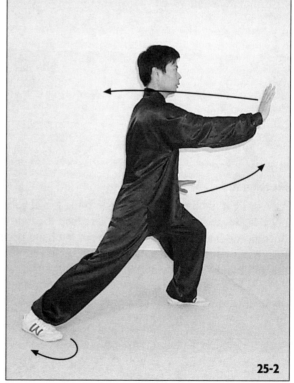

25-2

Movement 2

Turn your body to the left to 3 o'clock as you step your left foot to the 2 o'clock position to form a left bow stance. Shift your major weight onto your left leg. At the same time, curve your right forearm and push your right hand forward by the side of your right ear at nose level, with the palm facing forward. Bring your left hand down in a circular motion and brush past your left knee, coming to rest beside your left hip. Look at the fingertips of your right hand.

✔ Key Points

1. When your left foot steps out, push your right hand out as your body weight shifts forward. The right hand pushing depends more on the body movement than on the arm.

2. Keep a transverse distance of 12 inches between your heels in a bow stance to hold a firm balance and an easy energy flow.

3. Keep your body erect. Drop your shoulder and keep your elbows down. Relax your waist and hips.

4. The left arm moves in a clockwise circle and the right arm moves in a counter-clockwise circle. Remember, your body's turn initiates your arm's motion.

5. Face 3 o'clock in the final position.

✔ Self-Defense Application

Block your attacker's punches by using your right arm, moving down and to the left, and your left arm, moving up and to the right. Both blocks are energized by your waist, not your arms. Following the two blocks, step your left foot forward to push your attacker with your right palm.

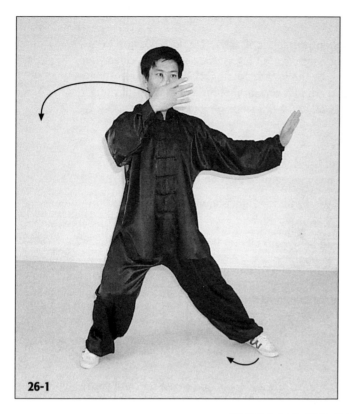

26-1

Movement 1

Rotate your right toes toward 6 o'clock, as you sit back and shift your body weight onto your right leg. Turn your body to the right, to 7 o'clock, with your left toes turning toward 6 o'clock. At the same time, move your right hand in a horizontal curve at shoulder level to your right side, with the right palm turning slowly outward and downward. Look at your right hand.

Posture 26

CROSS HANDS

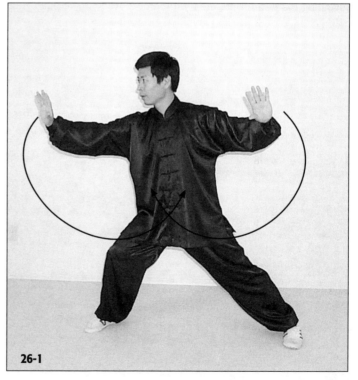

26-1

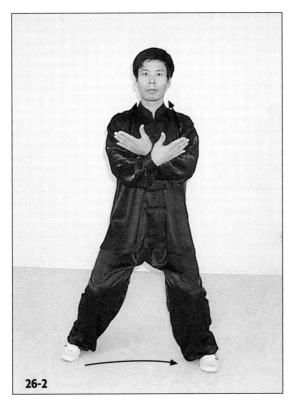

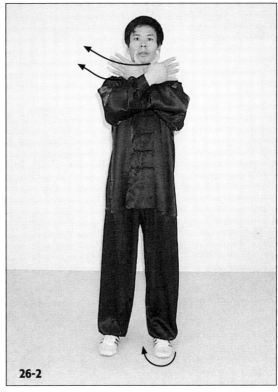

26-2

26-2

Movement 2

Shift your body weight slowly onto your left leg and bring your right foot toward your left foot, so they are parallel and a shoulder-width apart. Straighten both legs gradually and move both hands down in a vertical curve to cross at the wrist in front of your abdomen. Then move your hands up to shoulder level with your left hand nearer your body, palms facing inward. Look to the front. The arrows in the right photograph show the transition to Posture 27.

☑ Key Points

1. Place your weight evenly on both legs as your hands cross. Keep both arms in an arc shape, with elbows slightly bent.

2. Keep your body erect as you straighten your legs.

3. Face 6 o'clock in the final position.

☑ Self-Defense Application

As you sit back and turn to the left, pull and grab your right hand to deflect an attack. Bring both hands down in a circular motion and then up to protect your front body.

End of Sequence 2

It is optional to stop here, closing the form with Posture 74 (see page 226), or you can continue to practice with Sequence 3.

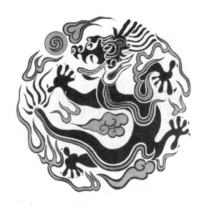

Sequence
3

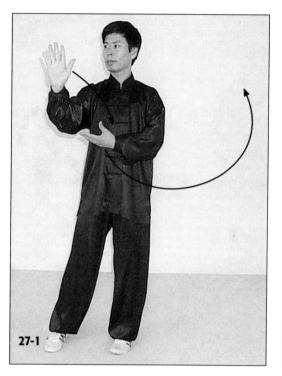

27-1

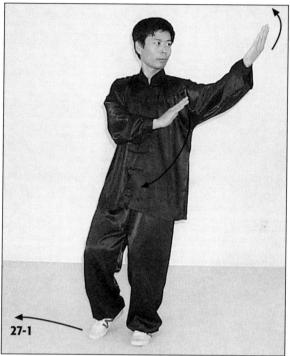

27-1

Posture 27

CARRY TIGER BACK TO MOUNTAIN

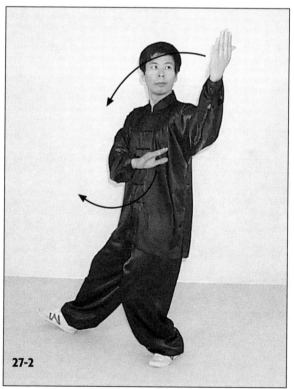

27-2

Movement 1

With your weight moving slightly to your right foot, turn your left toes in, then shift your weight onto your left leg. Bring your right foot back slightly, toes on the floor. Bend both legs slightly at the knees. At the same time, bring your left hand down to the left, then move it up in a curve to ear level with the palm facing obliquely upward. Move your right hand down in a curve in front of your body with the palm facing down. Look at your left hand.

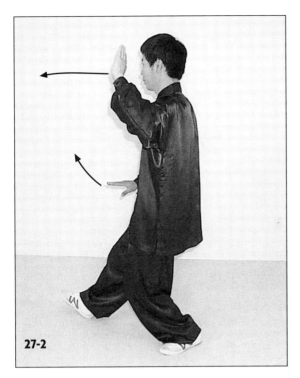

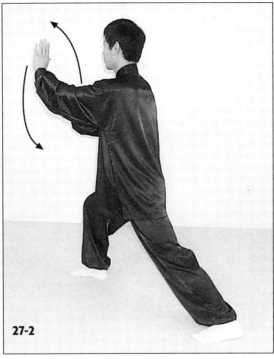

Movement 2

Turn your body to the right and step your right foot toward 10 o'clock to form a right bow stance. At the same time, bend your left forearm to push the palm out, with your fingers at nose level. Move your right hand in a downward curve across your abdomen, to the outside of your right knee at waist level, with the palm facing down. Look at your left hand.

☑ Key Points

1. Turn your body about 120 degrees to the right. After shifting your body weight onto your right leg, turn your left toes inward.

2. Pushing your left hand forward should be coordinated with forming a right bow stance and shifting your weight forward.

3. Keep your shoulders down and your upper body erect. This is the same as the Brush Knee posture, except that your right hand is slightly higher.

4. Face 10 o'clock in the final position.

☑ Self-Defense Application

Block an attacker's hand with your right hand, then step forward and push with your left hand. Keep your right hand higher, in order to intercept and grab an assailant's arm.

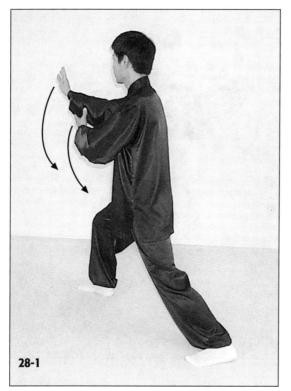

28-1

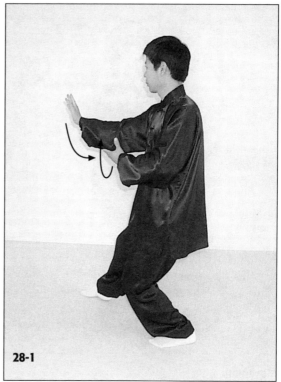

28-1

Posture 28

GRASP BIRD'S TAIL IN A DIAGONAL WAY

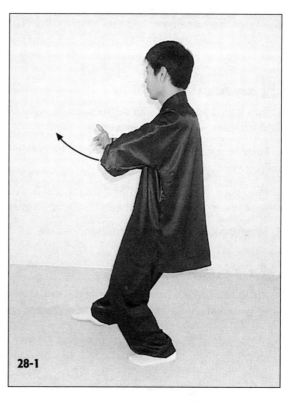

28-1

Movement 1

Raise your right hand to shoulder level and move your left hand back near your right elbow with the palm obliquely up. Turn your body slowly to the left, to 8 o'clock, and shift your weight onto your left leg. At the same time, pull both hands back, down and to the left, in a curve, with the left hand near your left hip, palm facing up.

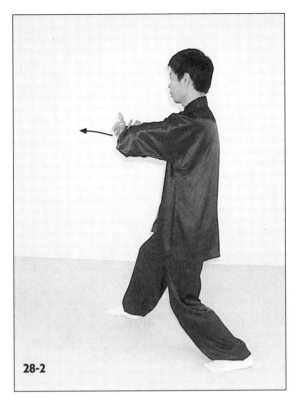

28-2

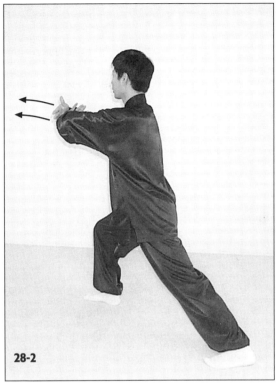

28-2

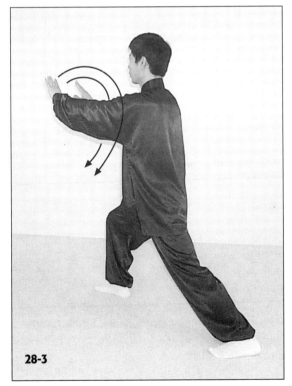

28-3

Movement 2

Turn your body slowly to the right, to 9 o'clock. Move your right hand toward your chest with palm facing obliquely inward. Turn your left palm down and move your left hand to the inside of your right wrist. Shift your body weight back to your right leg into a right bow stance while pressing both hands forward with your right palm facing inward and your left palm facing outward. Look at the right wrist.

Movement 3

Following the press out motion, separate your hands to a shoulder-width and turn both palms forward and down.

119

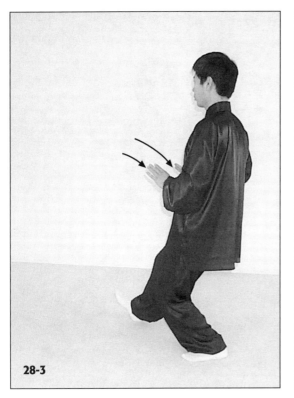

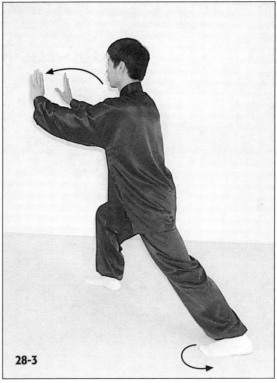

28-3

28-3

Sit back and shift your weight onto your left leg, raising up your right toes. At the same time, draw both hands back and down in a curve to the front of your abdomen, with the palms pressing down. Transfer your body weight slowly onto your right leg, while pushing both palms forward and upward in a curve to shoulder level. Bend your right knee to form a right bow stance. Look to the front.

☑ Key Points

1. Keep your waist and hips relaxed. Do not shrug your shoulders when pushing out your hands. Keep the elbows slightly down.

2. Coordinate your hands pushing with your body shifting forward. Use your body to generate the push instead of your arms.

3. Do not push your body weight too far forward. Your right knee should be behind your left toes.

4. Face 10 o'clock in the final position.

☑ Self-Defense Application

Grab your attacker's arm and pull it toward you by shifting your weight backward. Then, push out your right forearm by using the flow of your body weight shifting forward. Sit back and draw your hands back to avoid an attack. Then, pin your attacker's arms down and push toward his chest. Push upward and forward to destroy balance.

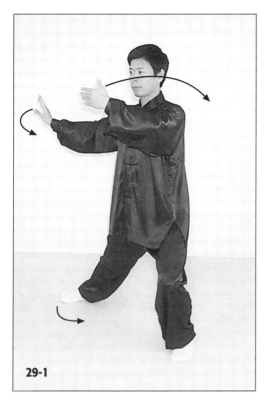

29-1

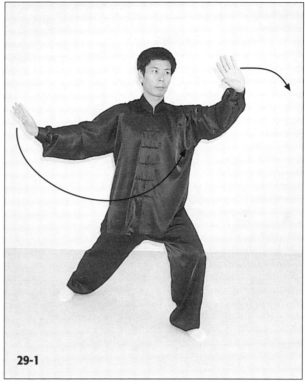

29-1

Posture 29

SINGLE WHIP

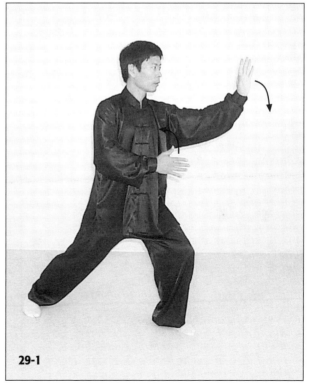

29-1

Movement 1

Rotate your left toes outward slightly as you sit back and shift your body weight gradually onto your left leg. Turn your right toes inward. Turn your body to the left, to 5 o'clock, and move your left hand back. Move both hands to the left, with your left hand on top and your right hand at abdomen level, until your left arm is extended sideways at shoulder level, with the palm turning outward. Bend your right arm at the elbow and curve your right hand up in front of your left ribs, with the palm facing obliquely inward and to the left. Look at your left hand.

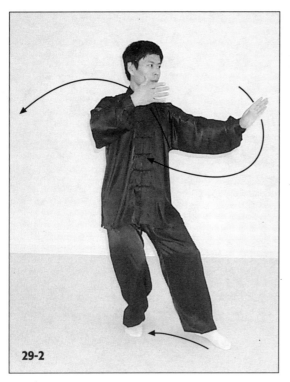

29-2

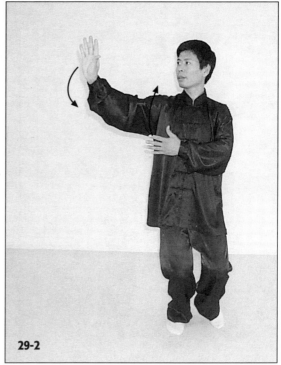

29-2

Movement 2

Shift your body weight slowly onto your right leg and turn your body to the right, to 7 o'clock. Bring your left foot back, next to your right foot, with its toes touching the ground. At the same time, move your right hand up in a curve to the upper side of your body. With palm turned outward, bunch your right fingertips and bend your wrist to form the hook of a bird beak. Move your left hand in a curve past your abdomen, up to the front of your right shoulder, with the palm facing inward.

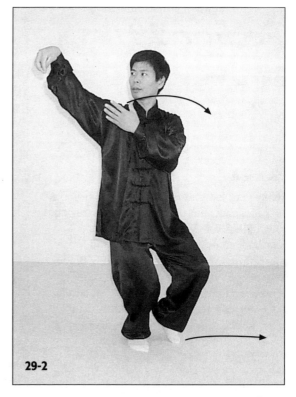

29-2

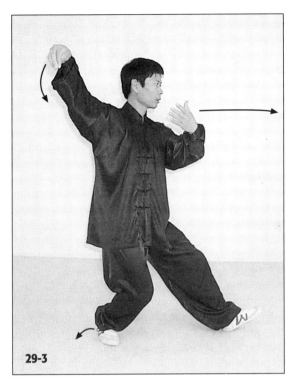

29-3

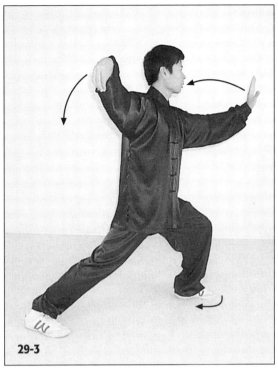

29-3

Movement 3

Turn your body to the left, to 4 o'clock. Step out with your left foot toward 2 o'clock. Shift your body weight onto your left leg to form a left bow stance. Turn your right heel outward slightly to make sure your toes are pointing to a position between 4 and 5 o'clock. At the same time, turn your left palm outward and push it out to the left, with its fingertips at eye level. Push and brace your right hooked hand toward 8 o'clock. Look at your left hand.

✅ Key Points

1. Mimic the motion of a whip. Swing your left arm out in coordination with turning your body.

2. Bend both arms slightly in the final position to keep your shoulders and elbows down. Your left elbow should be directly above your left knee.

3. As you push your left palm out, this should be synchronized with shifting your body weight forward to form the bow stance. The push is, therefore, powered by the body flow instead of the arm. Pushing energy comes from your feet, through your waist, and up to your left shoulder and arm.

4. Face 3 o'clock in the final position.

✅ Self-Defense Application

Move your arms in circles as your body and waist turn to block and intercept your attacker's hands. You can apply a splitting hit as you turn your palms outward. When stepping out and turning left, whip your left arm out like a strap to the left and then turn the palm to push and split your attacker's neck area.

123

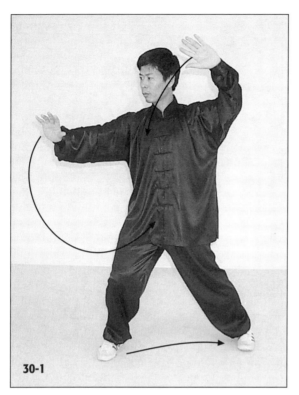

30-1

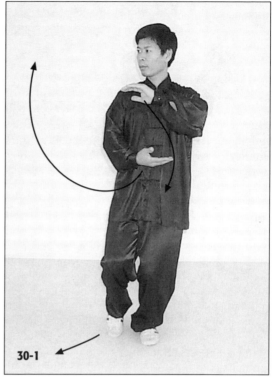

30-1

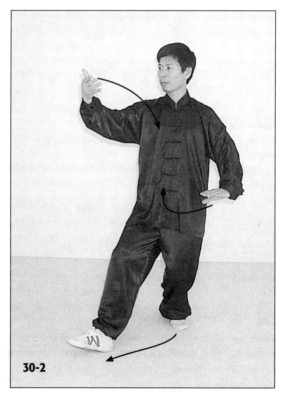

30-2

Posture 30

FAIR LADY WORKS WITH SHUTTLE—PUSH TO FOUR CORNERS

Movement 1

Sit back and shift your weight gradually onto your right leg, with your left toes turning inward. Turn your body to the right, to 6 o'clock, and move your left hand back in an upward curve to the side of your left ear. Open your right hooked hand and lower it. Then, shift your weight onto your left leg and bring your right foot back near your left, toes touching the floor. Move your left hand back in a downward curve to the front of your abdomen, palm facing up. At the same time, lower your right hand to shoulder level, palm facing down.

Movement 2

Turn your body to the right and step your right foot toward a position between 7 and 8 o'clock, toes turning outward. Bring your left foot near your right, toes touching the floor. At the same time, move your right hand up and to the right, then turn the palm down to lie in front of your right chest. Bring your left hand down and across your abdomen, bringing it to rest below your right hand with the palm facing up to form a hold-ball position.

Movement 3

Step your left foot toward a position between 7 and 8 o'clock and shift your weight onto your left leg to form a left bow stance. At the same time, raise your left hand in a curve past your face to lie above your forehead with the palm diagonally upward. Move your right hand back and down slightly, then push it forward and up to shoulder level. Face a position between 7 and 8 o'clock. Look at your right hand.

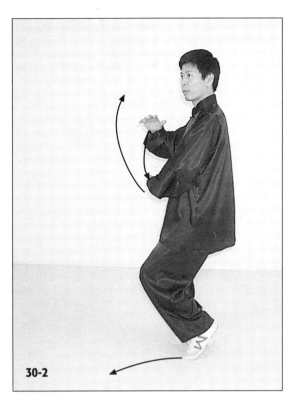

30-2

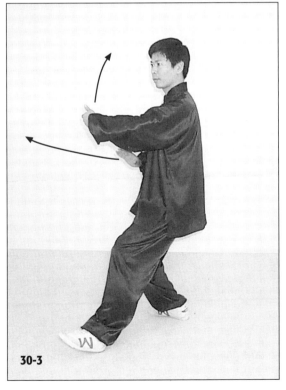

30-3

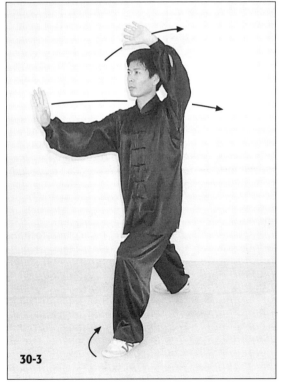

30-3

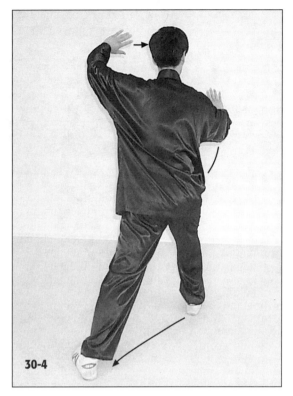

30-4

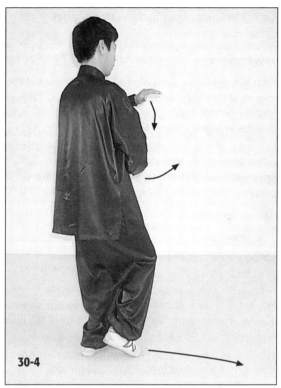

30-4

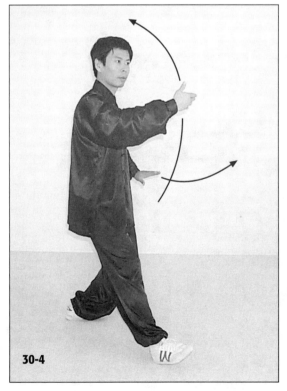

30-4

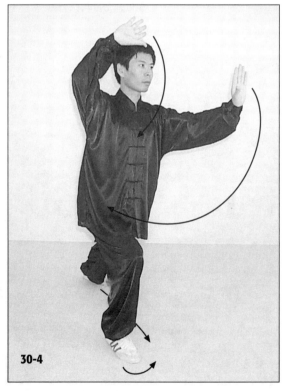

30-4

Movement 4

Rotate your right toes outward as you sit back. Then shift your weight onto your right leg, left toes turning inward. Shift your weight back to your left leg and turn your body about 180 degrees to the right, to 2 o'clock. Bring your right foot next to your left, toes touching the floor. Bring both hands back in curves to assume a hold-ball position in front of your left chest, with your left hand on top. Turn your body to the right an additional 90 degrees. Step your right foot toward a position between 4 and 5 o'clock and shift your weight onto your right leg to form a right bow stance. Raise your right hand in a curve past your face to lie above your forehead with the palm diagonally upward. Move your left hand back and slightly down, then push it forward and up to shoulder level. Face a position between 4 and 5 o'clock. Look at your left hand.

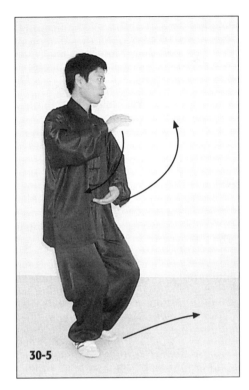

30-5

Movement 5

Shift your weight to your left leg and turn your right toes inward slightly. Then, shift your weight back to your right leg. Bring both hands back in curves to assume a hold-ball position in front of your right chest, with your right hand on the top. At the same time, turn your body slightly to the right and bring your left foot near your right. Step your left foot toward a position between 1 and 2 o'clock, and shift your weight onto your left leg to form a left bow stance. Meanwhile,

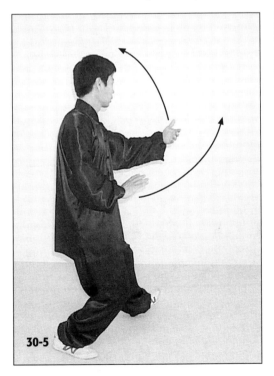

30-5

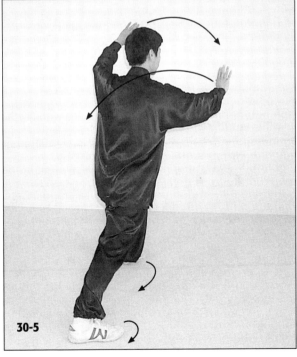

30-5

127

raise your left hand in a curve past your face to lie above your forehead with the palm diagonally upward. Move your right hand back and down slightly, then push it forward and up to shoulder level. Face a position between 1 and 2 o'clock. Look at your right hand.

Movement 6

Rotate your right toes outward as you sit back. Then shift your weight onto your right leg, left toes turning inward. Shift your weight back to your left leg and turn your body about 180 degrees to the right, to 7 o'clock. Bring your right foot next to your left, toes touching the floor. Bring both hands back in curves to assume a hold-ball position in front of your left chest, with your left hand on top. Turn your body to the right an additional 90 degrees. Step your right foot toward a position between 10 and 11 o'clock and shift your weight onto your right leg to form a right bow stance. Raise your right hand in a curve past your face to lie above your forehead with the palm diagonally upward. Move your left hand back and slightly down, then push it forward and up to shoulder level. Face a position between 10 and 11 o'clock. Look at your left hand.

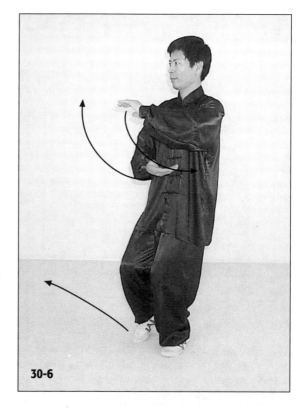

30-6

30-6

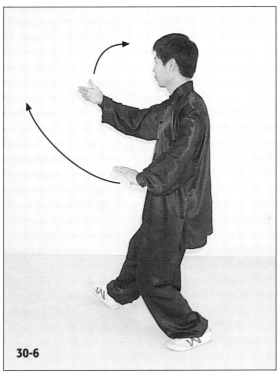

30-6

☑ Key Points

1. Like a fair lady who works a shuttle back and forth on a loom, you complete these movements by doing the same thing at the four oblique corners: front right; front left; back left, and back right.

2. Do not lift your shoulder when raising your hand above your forehead.

3. Coordinate your palm pushing forward with bending your front leg and shifting your weight forward.

4. When you step out to form a bow stance, keep a transverse distance of 12 inches between your heels for good balance and an easy energy flow.

5. Face a position between 10 and 11 o'clock in the final position.

☑ Self-Defense Application

This posture is useful when you are defending and fighting against multiple attackers from different directions. From a hold-ball position, lift your lower hand to intercept an attacker's punch, while stepping forward to strike the neck with the other hand. Imagine that you are weaving a shuttle back and forth and turning around to push the four oblique corners.

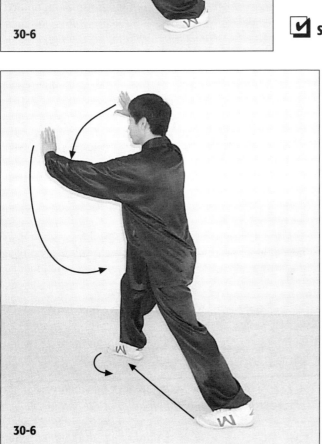

30-6

Posture 31

GRASP BIRD'S TAIL—LEFT

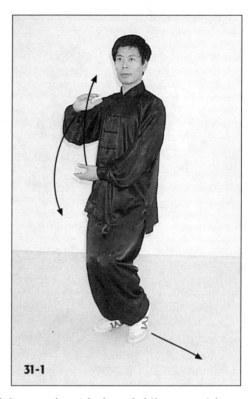

31-1

Movement 1

Shift your body weight onto your left leg and turn your body to the left, to 8 o'clock, right toes turning inward. Then, shift your weight back to your right leg and bring your left foot to the side of your right, placing its toes on the floor. Move your left hand to the left, down, and to the right, in a curve, past your abdomen, to make a hold-ball position, with your right hand in front of the right side of your chest.

Movement 2

Turn your body slightly to the left and step your left foot toward 5 o'clock. Continue turning your body to the left, toward 6 o'clock, and shift your weight onto your left leg to form a left bow stance. At the same time, move your left forearm up to shoulder level, your palm facing inward and your elbow bending as if warding off an attack. Drop your right hand to the side of your right hip, palm facing down. Look at your left forearm.

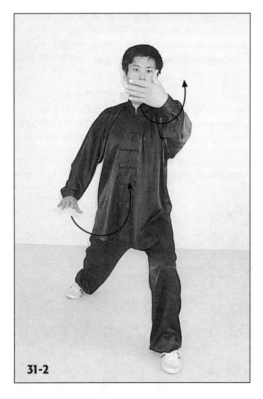

31-2

☑ Key Points

1. Make sure your left heel touches the floor first when taking the left step. As your body weight shifts forward, press your left sole down to make your whole left foot touch the floor.

2. Keep both arms rounded. Keep your shoulders and elbows sunk.

3. Coordinate your hand's separation with your body's turning and your left leg's bending.

4. Keep a 12-inch transverse distance between your feet when forming the bow stance.

5. Face 6 o'clock in the final position.

☑ Self-Defense Application

This is called the "Ward Off" movement. Use your left forearm to intercept your attacker's hand and dissolve the force by turning your body to the left. Bring your right arm down and lower your hand to protect yourself from your attacker's kick.

Grasp the Bird's Tail is composed of four techniques: ward off, roll back, press, and push. They are linked together to deflect an attack, and to pull or push an attacker off balance.

Movement 3

Turn your body slightly to the left, to a position between 5 and 6 o'clock, and extend your left hand forward, with the palm turning down as if grabbing something. Turn your right palm up and forward, and bring your right hand up across your abdomen until it is just below your left forearm. Then, turn your body slowly to the right, to 8 o'clock, and shift your weight back to your right leg. At the same time, pull both hands back, down, up, and to the right, in a curve,

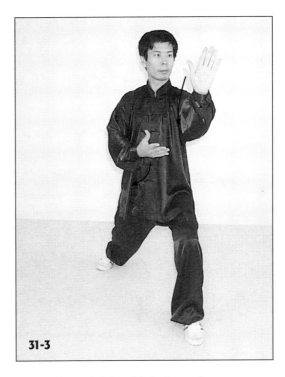

31-3

until your right hand is shoulder level with the palm facing up, and your left hand is in front of your chest with the palm facing inward. Your eyes should follow your right hand.

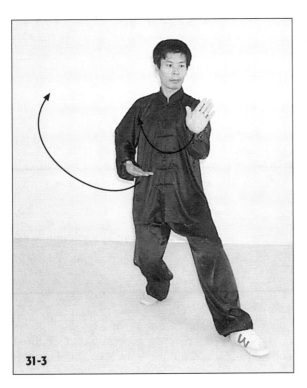

31-3

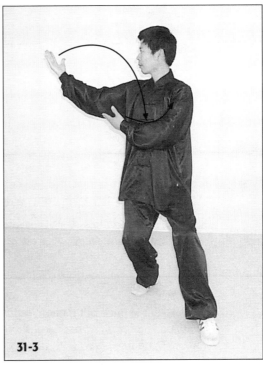

31-3

☑ Key Points

1. Pull back both arms in a circular movement as your body turns and your weight shifts back.

2. Keep your left foot flat on the floor. Do not lean your body forward or protrude your buttocks. Maintain your body in the center and root your feet into the ground to keep them solid and your body flexible.

3. Face 8 o'clock in the final position.

☑ Self-Defense Application

This is called a "Roll Back" movement. It allows you to hold your attacker's elbow and wrist to destroy balance. The pulling is energized through turning your waist and shifting your body weight backward.

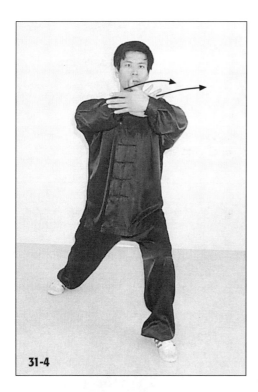

31-4

Movement 4

Turn your body slowly to the left, to 6 o'clock. Bend your right arm and bring your right hand to the inside of your left wrist. Shift your body weight to your left leg into a left bow stance while pressing both hands forward with your left palm facing inward and your right palm facing outward. Look at your left wrist.

☑ Key Points

1. Pressing your hands forward must be coordinated with your body turning and your weight shifting forward. The pressing force comes from your waist and spine, in addition to your body weight.

2. Keep both arms rounded and relaxed. Keep a 1-inch distance between your palms. Keep both shoulders sunk.

3. Keep your body erect. Do not lean forward when your hands press out. Keep both feet flat on the floor.

4. Face 6 o'clock in the final position.

☑ Self-Defense Application

This is called the "Press Out" movement. Use the flow of your body weight to press your left hand and forearm against your attacker's chest.

Movement 5

Following the press out motion, separate your hands to a shoulder-width and turn both palms forward and down. Sit back and shift your weight onto your right leg, raising up your left toes. At the same time, draw both hands back and down in a curve to the front of your abdomen,

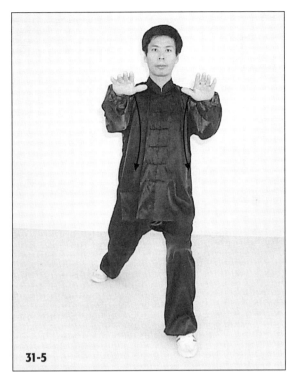

31-5

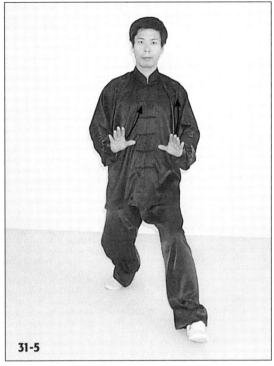

31-5

with the palms pressing down. Transfer your body weight slowly onto your left leg, while pushing both palms forward and upward in a curve to shoulder level. Bend your left knee to form a left bow stance. Look to the front. Arrows in bottom photograph show transition to Posture 32.

✔ Key Points

1. Keep your waist and hips relaxed. Do not shrug your shoulders when pushing out your hands. Keep your elbows slightly down.

2. Coordinate your hands pushing with your body shifting forward. Use your body to generate the push instead of your arms.

3. Do not push your body weight too far forward. Your left knee should be behind your left toes.

4. Face 6 o'clock in the final position.

✔ Self-Defense Application

This is called the "Push Out" movement. Sit back and draw your hands back to avoid an attack. Then, pin your attacker's arms down and push toward his chest. Push upward and forward to destroy balance.

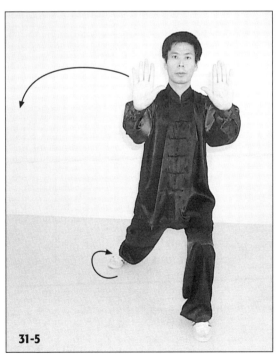

31-5

Posture 32

TURN AND KICK WITH RIGHT HEEL

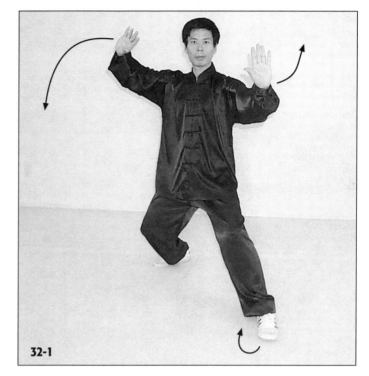

32-1

Movement 1

Turn your body to the right, to 9 o'clock, pivot your right foot outward, and shift your weight onto your right leg. Then turn your left toes inward. Move your right hand to the right in a downward curve, palm rotating outward.

Movement 2

Shift your weight back to your left leg and bring your right foot next to your left. Continue to move your right hand down, to the left and up, in a circular motion, while moving your left hand up and to the right in a curve, then down in front of your chest, crossing inside your right hand.

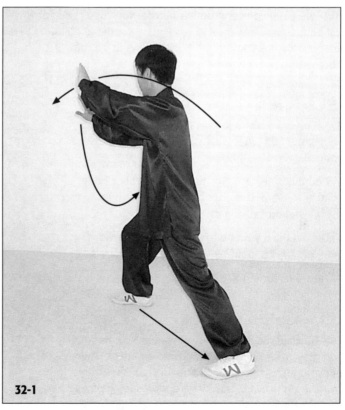

32-1

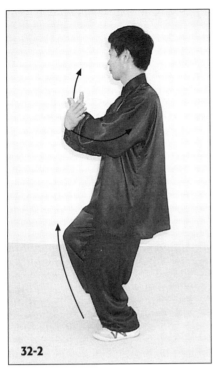

32-2

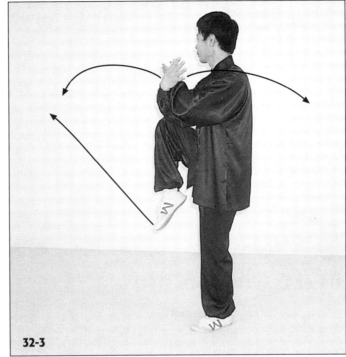

32-3

Movement 3

Lift your right foot and start to rotate both palms, separating them to your sides. At the same time, extend and kick out your right heel, toward a position between 10 and 11 o'clock. Your right hand should be just above your right leg, and your left hand should be extended to your left side. Look at your right hand. Arrows in bottom photograph show transition to Posture 33.

✔ Key Points

1. Do not lean your upper body forward or back. Keep your body in firm balance.

2. Separating your hands should be synchronized with kicking out your right heel. Extend your hands horizontally on both sides of your body at shoulder level, palms facing out.

3. Your supporting left leg should be straightened, but not locked, as you kick out your right heel.

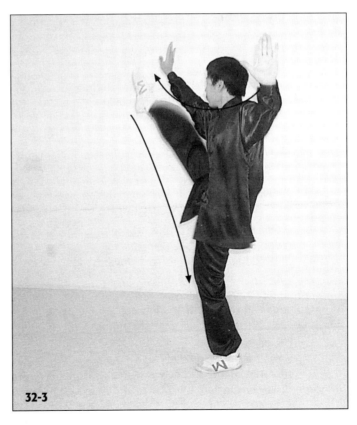

32-3

4. Your right arm and leg should be aligned vertically.

5. Face 9 o'clock in the final position.

☑ Self-Defense Application

Use your right forearm to intercept an attacker's punch and lift your right foot to kick the upper body with your heel. Keep your right hand above your right leg to protect against being grabbed. You can also kick the attacker's ribs or abdomen area if you cannot kick higher.

Posture 33

HIT EARS WITH BOTH FISTS

Movement 1

Turn your body to the right, to a position between 10 and 11 o'clock, and bend your right leg at the knee. Hold your thigh parallel to the ground and keep your right toes pointing downward. Move your left hand in a curve closer to your right hand, with both palms facing up. Look to the front.

Movement 2

Lower your hands to abdomen level, while stepping down your right foot toward a position between 10 and 11 o'clock. Shift your weight forward onto your right leg to make a right bow stance. Change your hands into fists and circle both fists forward, up, and in to form a pincer shape in front of you at head level, with fist eyes facing obliquely downward. Keep a distance of 6 inches between your fists. Look at your fists.

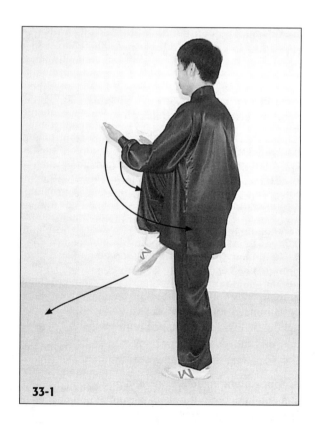

33-1

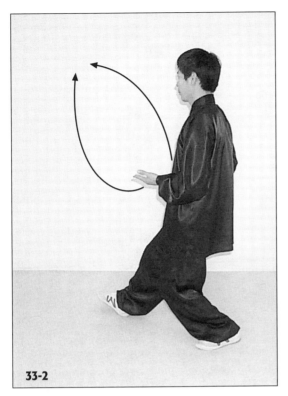

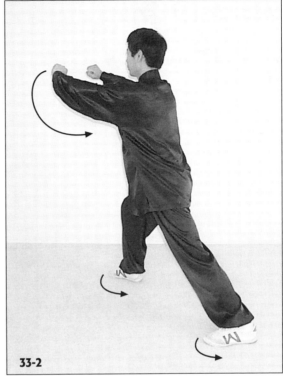

33-2

33-2

Key Points

1. Keep your chest and waist relaxed and hold your head and neck upright. Keep your shoulders sunk and elbows dropped.

2. Keep both arms in an arc shape. Hold your fists loosely.

3. Hitting out your fists should follow your body shifting forward.

4. Face a position between 10 and 11 o'clock in the final position.

☑ Self-Defense Application

Push an attacker's hands downward and out, then step forward to hit the temples with your fists, swinging from both sides.

Posture 34

TURN AND KICK WITH LEFT HEEL

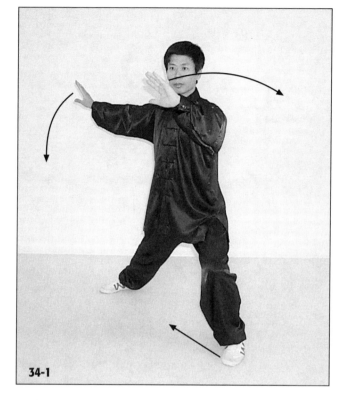

34-1

Movement 1

Rotate your left toes outward as you turn your body to the left, to 7 o'clock. Shift your weight onto your left leg and turn your right toes inward. Open your fists and separate them, moving them in a curve to both sides of your body. Your eyes should follow your left hand.

Movement 2

Shift your weight back onto your right leg. Lift up your left foot, toes pointing down. Move both hands down, in, and up, in a curve, crossing your palms in front of your chest, with your right hand outside.

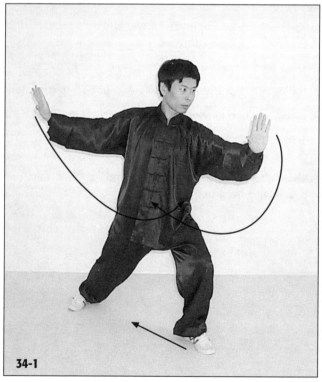

34-1

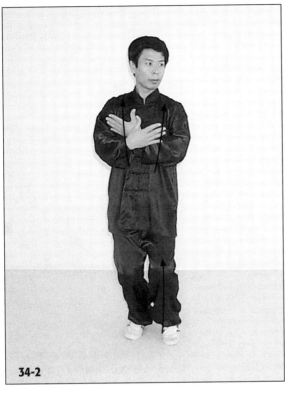

34-2

Movement 3

Rotate and separate your palms, extending both arms with palms facing outward. Kick your left heel out above waist level toward a position between 4 and 5 o'clock.

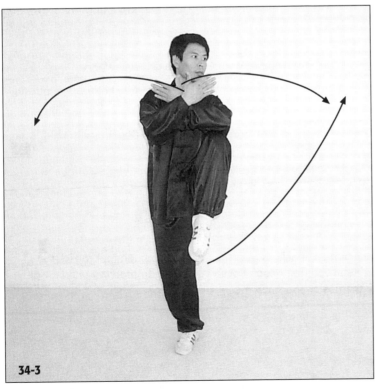

34-3

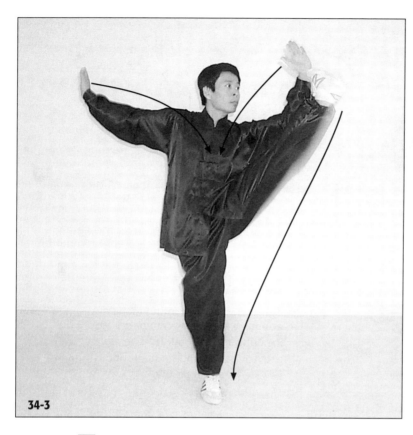

34-3

Your left hand should be just above your left leg. Look at your left hand. Arrows show transition to Posture 35.

☑ Key Points

1. Do not lean your upper body forward or back. Keep your body in firm balance.

2. Separating your hands should be synchronized with kicking out your right heel. Extend your hands horizontally on both sides of your body to shoulder level, with palms facing out.

3. Your supporting left leg should be straightened, but not locked, as you kick out your right heel.

4. Your right arm and leg should be aligned vertically.

5. Face 6 o'clock in the final position.

☑ Self-Defense Application

Use your left forearm to intercept an attacker's punch and lift up your left foot to kick the upper body with your heel. Keep your left hand above your left leg to protect against being grabbed. You can also kick the ribs or abdomen area if you cannot kick higher.

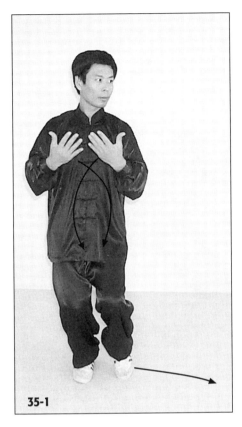

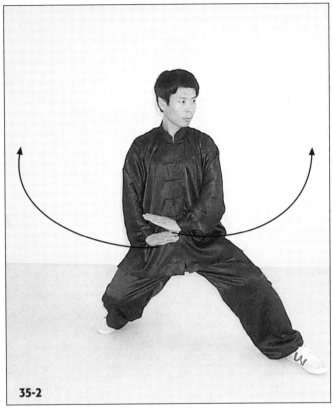

35-1

35-2

Posture 35

COVER HAND AND THRUST FIST

Movement 1

Bring your left foot back, toes touching the floor next to your right foot. Pull your arms close to each other in front of your chest, palms facing inward.

Movement 2

Turn your chest to the right slightly as you step your left foot toward 3 o'clock, with the inner side of your left heel scraping along the floor. At the same time, turn both palms facing down and cross them. Press both palms down in front of your abdomen with your left hand on top.

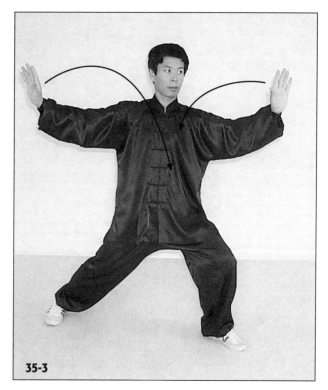

35-3

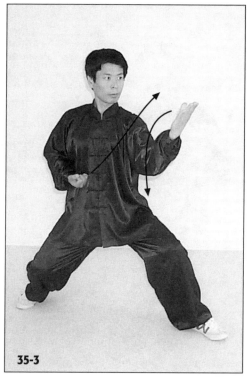

35-3

35-4

Movement 3

Shift your weight onto your left leg slightly to form a half horse-riding stance. At the same time, separate your hands and move them up on both sides of your body, then forward to the front of your chest. Clench your right hand into a fist and hide it inside your left forearm. Look to the front.

Movement 4

Turn your body swiftly to the left to 4 o'clock, with your right leg straightened to form a left bow stance. At the same time, thrust your right fist straight forward, to 6 o'clock, at chest level, while withdrawing your left hand to your left side, with the palm gently touching your left abdomen. Look at your right fist. Arrow shows transition to Posture 36.

☑ Key Points

1. It is typical of the Chen Tai Chi style to combine soft and slow motions with a sud-

den quick tempo. Chen style emits power like an arrow coming off a bow. Arch your back and store up the energy before thrusting your right fist.

2. Thrusting out your right fist should be coordinated with your body's swift turning.

3. Face 5 o'clock in the final position.

☑ Self-Defense Application

Press and deflect an attacker's hand, then thrust your right fist onto the chest. Do it in a quick tempo.

Posture 36

SPLIT PALMS IN A HORSE-RIDING STANCE

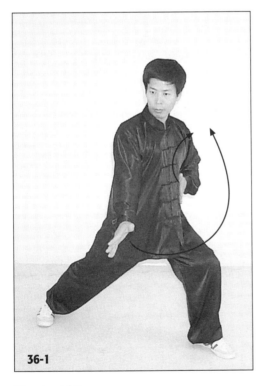

36-1

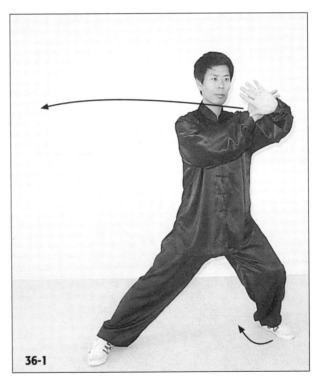

36-1

Movement 1

While twisting your upper body, open your right fist and swing your right hand in a clockwise circle to the front of your left shoulder. Shift your weight to your left leg and raise your left hand to the inside of your right forearm. Overlap your hands to form a circle in front of your left chest, right palm facing inward, left palm facing outward. Look at both hands.

143

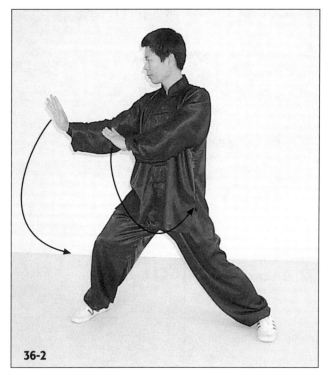

36-2

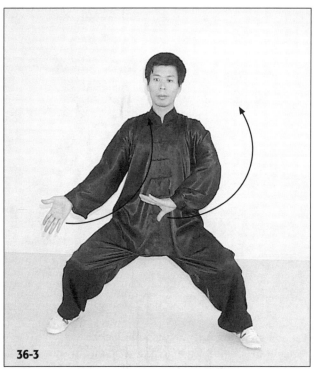

36-3

Movement 2

Without any pause, turn your body to the right, to 8 o'clock, and swing both hands in a curve to the right, with your right palm rotating outward. Your eyes should follow both hands.

Movement 3

Turn your body slightly to the left, to 6 o'clock and distribute your weight evenly on both feet to form a horse-riding stance. At the same time, move both hands down in a curve along your right side. Then, pull your left hand to the front of your abdomen, and your right hand to the top of your right knee. Rotate and split both palms toward 5 o'clock.

☑ Key Points

1. This is another popular posture of the Chen Tai Chi style. Twist your waist to lead your arms' swing around your body, with your palms rotating outward, and apply a splitting power.

2. Keep both feet rooted to the ground when you stand in the horse-riding stance.

3. Face 6 o'clock in the final position.

☑ Self-Defense Application

Intercept an attacker's hand with your right hand, and grab the arm to pull it to your rear right side. Twist your waist to the left with both palms splitting into the lower body.

Posture 37

STAND ON ONE LEG TO PUNCH TIGER

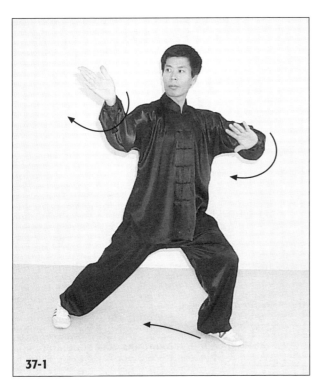

37-1

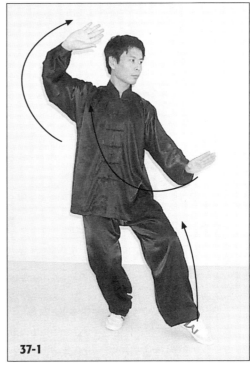

37-1

Movement 1

Turn your body to the left, to 4 o'clock, and shift your weight to your left leg. Swing both arms up, slightly back, and to the left, so that each hand draws a small circle in front of your left chest. Shift your weight back to your right leg, left toes touching the floor. Swing both arms down and to the right in a curve, with both palms rotating outward.

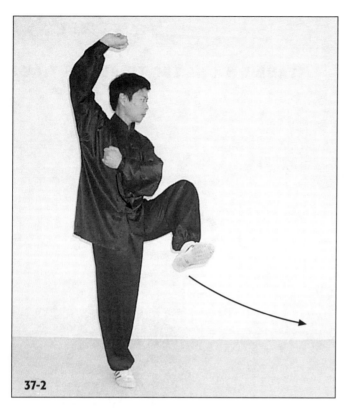

37-2

Movement 2

Continue circling both arms, moving your right hand above your head at the side of your right temple. Clench it into a fist with the fist eye facing obliquely inward. Move your left hand to the front of your right ribs, with the back of the fist facing outward. Stand on your right leg and raise your left leg with the knee fully bent. The bottom of your left foot should turn inward with toes slightly upward. Look at a 3 o'clock position.

✔ Key Points

1. This is a Wu-style Tai Chi posture. When you stand on your right leg, your left toes should be bent upward instead of pointing downward, as in the Yang style.

2. Keep your right knee slightly bent. Hold up your left knee as high as possible, so that your left foot can protect your crotch area.

3. Keep both arms in a curved shape. Do not bring your left arm too close to your body.

4. Face 5 o'clock in the final position.

✔ Self-Defense Application

Swing both arms to fend off an attacker's punch. Hold your fists to protect your head and rib area. Lift your left foot to block your crotch and prepare to kick your attacker's knee.

Posture 38

SQUAT DOWN TO PENETRATE LEFT FIST

Movement 1

Squat down slowly as far as your right knee can bend and extend your left leg straight out to the left, to 3 o'clock. Keep your left leg close to the floor, toes turning inward.

Movement 2

Turn your body slightly to the left, to 4 o'clock. Move your left fist down to your left thigh. Then slide your fist forward along the inside of your left leg until it is next to your left foot, with the fist eye facing upward. Extend your right fist outward, to 8 o'clock, turning the fist eye up. Look at your left fist. Arrows in bottom photograph show transition to Posture 39.

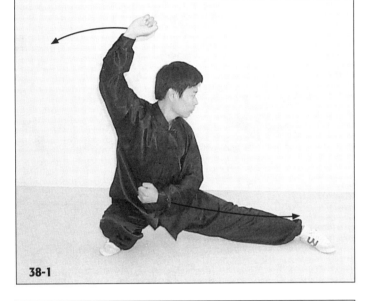

38-1

✔ Key Points

1. When you squat down, do not let your upper body lean too far forward. Practice lowering your body gradually. Go as low as you can without discomfort.

2. Your bent right knee should point in the same direction as your toes to prevent it from being twisted.

3. Try to stretch your left leg straight out and close to the floor. Keep your left foot fully touching the floor.

4. Face 4 o'clock in the final position.

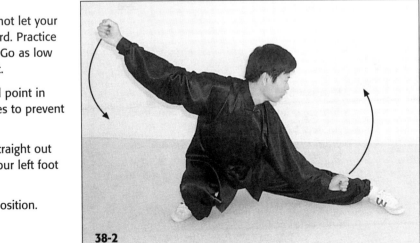

38-2

✔ Self-Defense Application

Squatting down to lower your body is a defensive movement to avoid an attacker's high attack. At the same time, you can extend and stretch your left leg forward, and with your left arm under the legs, you can throw an attacker off balance.

147

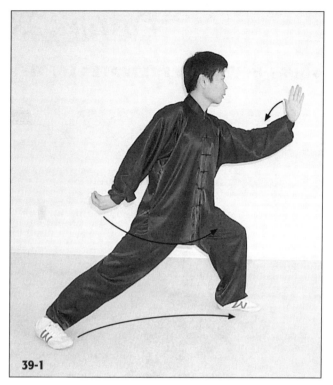

39-1

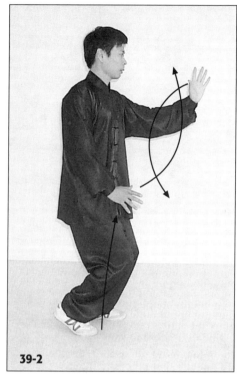

39-2

Posture 39

GOLDEN ROOSTER STANDS
ON ONE LEG—LEFT

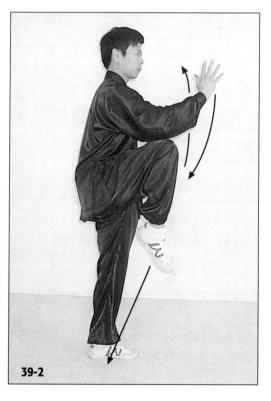

39-2

Movement 1

Turn your left toes forward and your body to the left, to 3 o'clock. Shift your weight forward onto your left leg to form a left bow stance. Open both fists and move your left hand up and forward to shoulder level, lowering your right palm behind you into a hook-hand position, fingers pointing obliquely up. Look at your left hand.

Movement 2

Slowly lift your right leg, with knee fully bent and toes pointing downward. At the same time, open your right hook-hand and move it forward and up to shoulder level, with your elbow above your right knee and your palm facing left. Lower your left hand to the side of your hip, with the palm facing down and fingers pointing forward. Look at your right hand.

☑ Key Points

1. Your left leg should be slightly bent to ensure solid balance while standing on one leg. Keep your upper body upright and steady.

2. When you lift your right leg, imagine that your right hand is pulling the leg up, as if you were a puppet.

3. Keep your right foot relaxed, with the toes pointing downward.

4. Face 3 o'clock in the final position.

☑ Self-Defense Application

Press your left palm down to deflect an attacker's hand and move your right hand forward to spear it up. When you lift your right leg, you can hit an assailant with your right knee while setting yourself up in a kicking position.

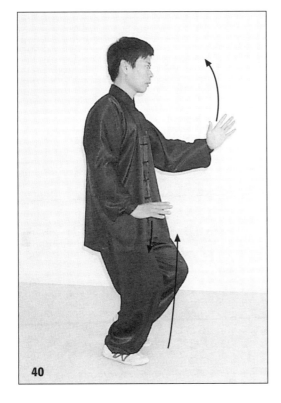

40

Posture 40

GOLDEN ROOSTER STANDS ON ONE LEG–RIGHT

Step your right foot down beside your left, toes turning outward slightly. Then, shift your weight onto it. Slowly lift your left leg, with the knee fully bent and toes pointing downward. At the same time, bring your left hand up to shoulder level so that your elbow is above your left knee, palm facing right. Lower your right hand to the side of your right hip, with the palm facing down and fingers pointing forward. Look at your left hand. Arrows in top photograph on page 150 show transition to Posture 41.

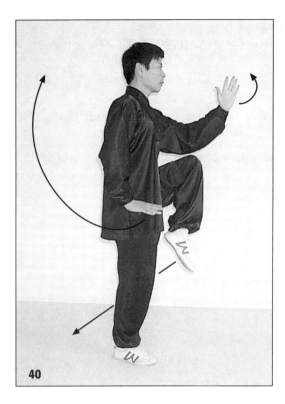

40

Key Points

1. Your right leg should be slightly bent to ensure solid balance while standing on one leg. Keep your upper body upright and steady.

2. When you lift your left leg, imagine that your left hand is pulling the leg up, as if you were a puppet.

3. Keep your left foot relaxed, with the toes pointing downward.

4. Face 3 o'clock in the final position.

Self-Defense Application

Press your right palm down to deflect an attacker's hand and move your left hand forward to spear it up. When you lift your left leg, you can hit an assailant with your left knee while setting yourself up in a kicking position.

Posture 41

REPULSE MONKEY

Movement 1

Step your left foot back toward 10 o'clock and turn your body to the right, to 5 o'clock. Bring your right hand back in a curve past your right thigh and up to shoulder level, with the palm rotating up. At the same time, turn your left palm up, fingers pointing forward.

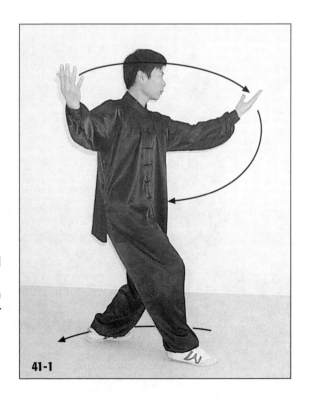

41-1

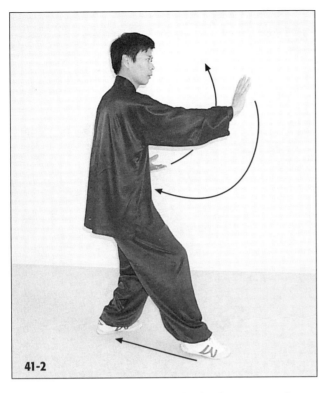

41-2

Movement 2

Turn your body to the left, to 2 o'clock. Bend your right elbow and push your right palm forward by the side of your right ear, fingers pointing up. Shift your weight onto your left foot to form a right empty stance with your right foot straight up, facing 3 o'clock. At the same time, lower your left hand to the side of your left waist, palm facing up.

✔ Key Points

1. Keep your arms in curve when pushing out or drawing back your palms. Do not lock your elbows.

2. When stepping back, place your toes down first, then gradually shift your weight back and make your whole foot touch the floor. When shifting your weight back, pivot on your front toes to make them point forward.

3. Keep your waist and hips relaxed. Move your foot a little sideways as you step back to prevent locking your hips.

4. Keep your eyes on the movement of your active hand. When your palms cross each other in front of your chest, try to sense the magnetic repulsion between them.

5. Face 3 o'clock in the final position.

✔ Self-Defense Applications

Use your front hand to intercept or grab an attacker's arm. Step back to pull an attacker over. Strike out with the other hand toward your attacker's head or chest.

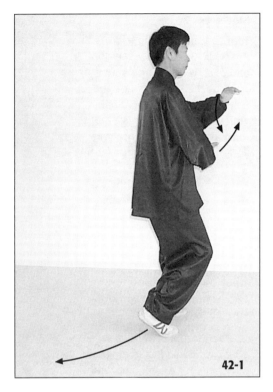

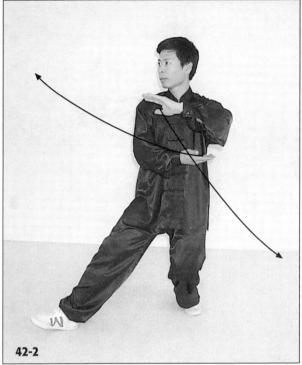

42-1

42-2

Posture 42

DIAGONAL FLY

Movement 1

Move your right hand down in a curve to the front of your left ribs, palm turning upward. At the same time, move your left hand up in a curve from your rear left to the front of your left chest, palm turning downward to form a hold-ball position. Bring your right foot next to your left, toes touching the floor.

Movement 2

Turn your body to the right, to 5 o'clock, and step your right foot to 8 o'clock. Shift your weight onto your right leg. At the same time, separate your hands, with the right hand moving up and to the right slightly higher than your head with the palm facing obliquely upward. Your left hand descends to the side of your left hip, palm facing obliquely down and fingers pointing forward. Lean your right shoulder toward 8 o'clock. Look to your left.

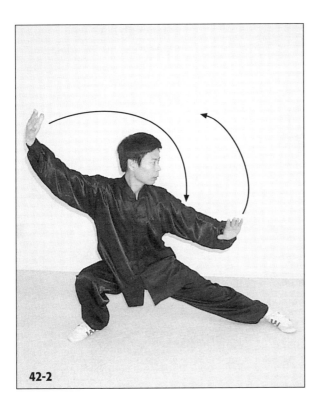

42-2

☑ Key Points

1. This is a popular Wu-style posture. Turn your body smoothly to the right for a good balance.

2. Coordinate extending your right arm outward with forming the right-side bow stance.

3. Lean your upper body to the right, but do not lean too far. This is called "tilted upright" in the Wu style.

4. Face 5 o'clock in the final position.

☑ Self-Defense Application

To fight an attacker behind you, step your right foot back to get closer. Use your waist-turning power to throw your right arm and shoulder forward. Knock your attacker off balance in a spinning motion.

Posture 43

SQUAT DOWN TO PENETRATE RIGHT PALM

Movement 1

Shift your weight and turn your body to the left slightly. Then, bend your left knee and straighten your right leg to form a left-side bow stance. At the same time, move your right arm across your face to the left, bringing it to rest in front of your left chest. Raise your left hand toward 3 o'clock at head level, with your fingers held together into a hook-hand.

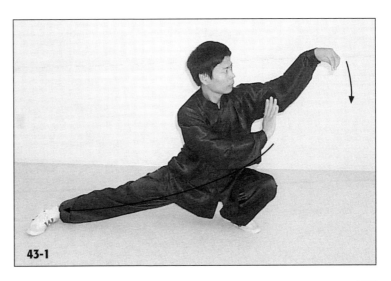

43-1

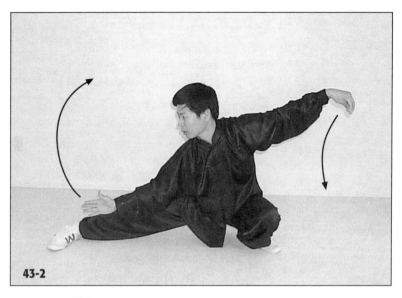

43-2

Movement 2

Squat down on your left leg and extend your right leg as far as you can to the right, right toes turning inward. At the same time, move your right hand down and extend it along the inside edge of your right leg, until it is next to your right foot. Look at your right hand. Arrows show transition to Posture 44.

✔ Key Points

1. When you squat down, do not let your upper body lean too far forward. Practice lowering your body gradually. Go as low as you can without discomfort.

2. Your bent left knee should point in the same direction as your toes to prevent it from being twisted.

3. Try to stretch your right leg straight out and close to the floor. Keep your right foot fully touching the floor.

4. Face 8 o'clock in the final position.

✔ Self-Defense Application

Squatting down to lower your body is a defensive movement to avoid an attacker's high attack. At the same time, you can extend and stretch your right leg forward and with your right arm under the legs, throw the attacker off balance.

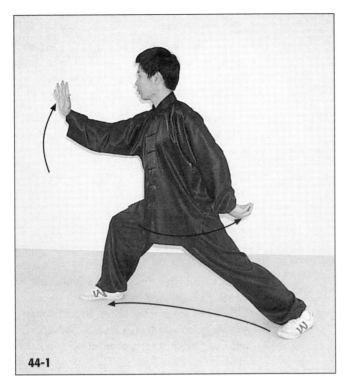

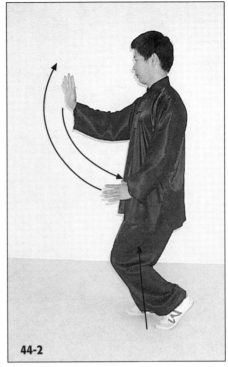

44-1

44-2

Posture 44

GOLDEN ROOSTER STANDS ON ONE LEG–RIGHT

Movement 1

Turn your right toes forward and your body to the right to 9 o'clock. Shift your weight forward onto your right leg to form a right bow stance. Move your right hand up and forward to shoulder level, lowering your left hook-hand behind you, fingers pointing obliquely up. Look at your right hand.

Movement 2

Slowly lift your left leg, with knee fully bent and toes pointing downward. At the same time, open your left hook-hand and move it forward and up to shoulder level with your elbow above your left knee and your palm facing left. Lower your right hand to your side hip, with the palm facing down and fingers pointing forward. Look at your left hand.

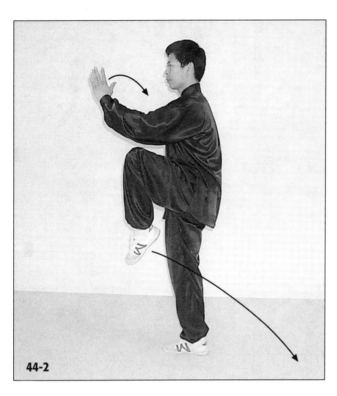

44-2

Key Points

1. Your right leg should be slightly bent to ensure solid balance while standing on one leg. Keep your upper body upright and steady.

2. When you lift your left leg, imagine that your left hand is pulling the leg up, as if you were a puppet.

3. Keep your left foot relaxed, with the toes pointing downward.

4. Face 9 o'clock in the final position.

Self-Defense Application

Press your right palm down to deflect an attacker's hand and move your left hand forward to spear it up. When you lift your left leg, you can hit an assailant with your left knee while setting yourself up in a kicking position.

Posture 45

STEP BACK AND SPEAR RIGHT PALM

Turn your left palm down and lower it to chest level. Step back with your left foot toward 4 o'clock to form a right bow stance. Press your left palm down and pull it closer to your body, while spearing out your right palm over your left forearm at neck level. Rotate your right palm up as you spear it forward. Look at your right hand.

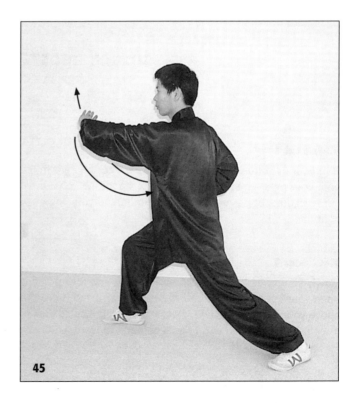

45

☑ Key Points

1. Step back to form a bow stance, popular in the typical Wu style. Spear your hand forward as you step your leg back.

2. Keep your shoulders sunk and your upper body erect.

3. Face 9 o'clock in the final position.

☑ Self-Defense Application

Step your left leg back to set up a firm bow stance. Lower your left palm to block an attacker's arm. Grab and pull the arm down and thrust your right palm from your waist with your fingers pointing toward your attacker's neck.

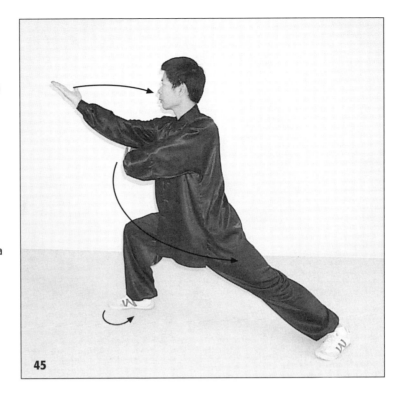

45

46-1

Posture 46

WILD HORSE THROWS ITS HOOF

Movement 1

Shift your weight to your left leg and turn your body to the left, to 4 o'clock. At the same time, bend your right arm at the elbow and turn your forearm, positioned vertically, all the way to the right, while moving your left hand down to the side of your left hip, palm facing down. Look at your right hand.

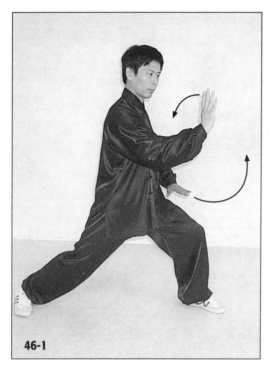

46-1

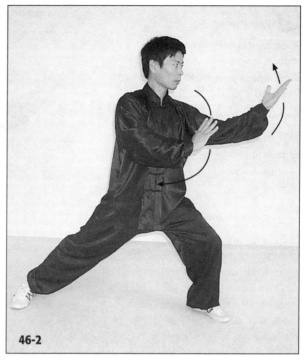

46-2

Movement 2

Without any pause, shift your weight back to your right leg and turn your body to the right, to 8 o'clock. Bring your left palm up in a circular motion from outside and bend your left arm at the elbow. Let your left forearm, positioned vertically, turn all the way to the left, while moving your right hand down to the side of your right hip, palm facing down. Look at your left hand.

Movement 3

Turn your body to the left, to 6 o'clock, and bend both knees to form a horse-riding stance. Move your left palm down and to the left across your abdomen, bringing it to rest above your left knee, palm facing down and slightly out. At the same time, throw your right hand up and forward at chest level, with

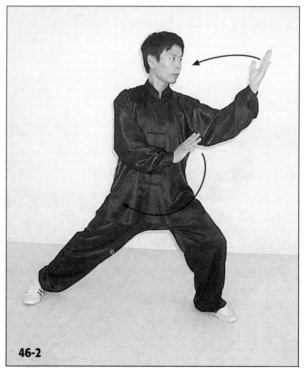

46-2

your palm facing up and slightly forward. Look at your right hand.

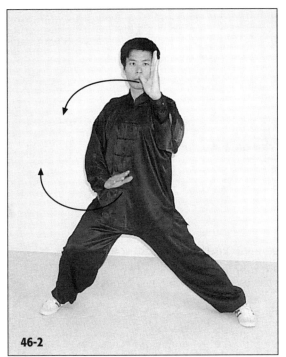

46-2

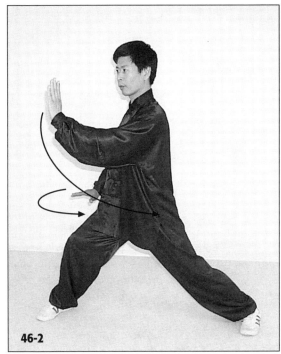

46-2

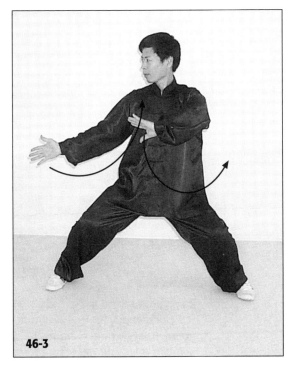

46-3

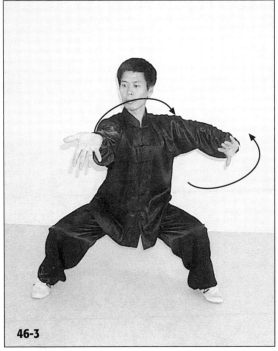

46-3

☑ Key Points

1. Stand with your feet about two shoulder widths apart. Bend both knees and keep your back straight, tucking your sacrum in slightly. Distribute your weight evenly on both feet.

2. Keep your feet parallel, toes pointing in the same direction as your chest. You may turn your toes outward slightly when you stand in a wider horse stance.

3. Twist your waist, letting both arms swing in front of your body.

4. This is modified from the Chen style. You may do it in a quick tempo when you split your right palm forward.

5. Face 6 o'clock in the final position.

☑ Self-Defense Application

Both arms should take turns swinging in large vertical circles in front of your body to block punches. Throw your right palm up toward an attacker's lower body to lift and destroy balance. Your upward push should be energized by your body power, not by your arm.

Posture 47

PART WILD HORSE'S MANE–LEFT

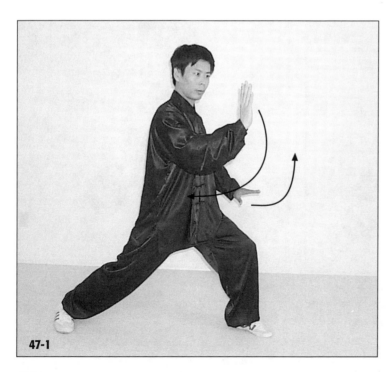

47-1

Movement 1

Turn your body to the left to 4 o'clock, and shift your weight to your left leg to form a left bow stance. Move your right arm up and to the left in a curve, to the front of your left shoulder. Look at your right hand.

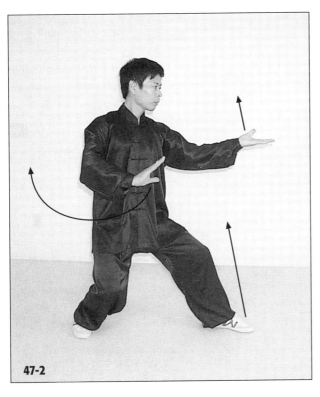

47-2

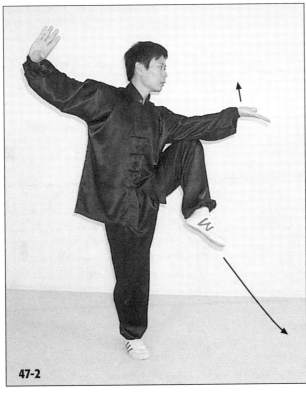

47-2

Movement 2

Shift your weight onto your right leg and turn your body to the right, to 5 o'clock. At the same time, move your right hand down in front of your chest, with the palm rotating down and out, while moving your left hand in a small counterclockwise circle at the outside of your left thigh. Without any pause, straighten your right knee and lift your left leg with the knee bent. Move your right hand up to your rear right side, at shoulder level, with the palm facing out. Move your left hand up at the same time, bringing it to rest above your left knee at shoulder level, palm rotating up. Look at your left palm.

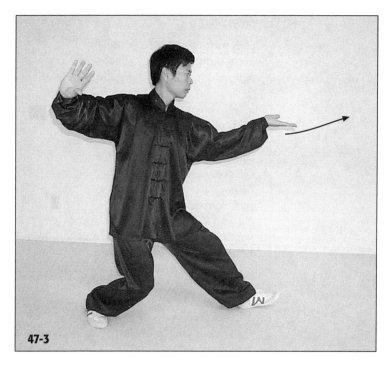

47-3

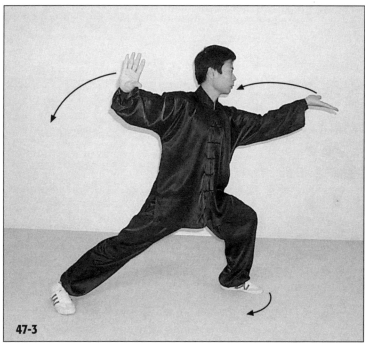

47-3

Movement 3

Bend your right leg to squat down and step your left foot out to 2 o'clock, heel scraping along the floor. Shift your weight forward onto your left leg to form a left bow stance. Stretch your left hand explosively forward to 3 o'clock, with the palm facing up and slightly forward. Look at your left hand.

☑ Key Points

1. Part Wild Horse's Mane in the Chen style is different from the Yang style. Always twist your waist and upper body to start a major motion in the Chen style.

2. Keep both palms rotating when swinging your arms around your body.

3. It is optional to form a half horse-riding stance instead of a bow stance in the final position.

4. Face 3 o'clock in the final position.

☑ Self-Defense Application

Intercept an attacker's punch with your right hand and deflect the arm toward your rear right. Put your left foot behind your attacker's leg to lock it and gain control. Stretch your left arm under the armpit and tumble your assailant down with your arm and shoulder.

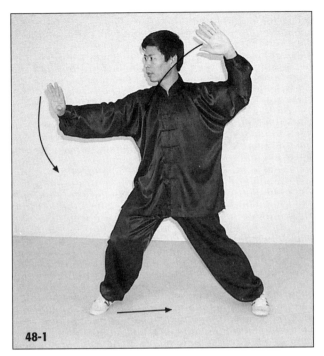

48-1

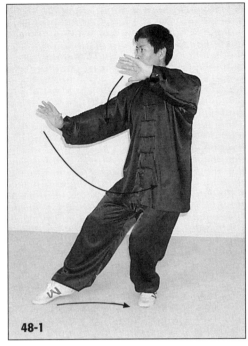

48-1

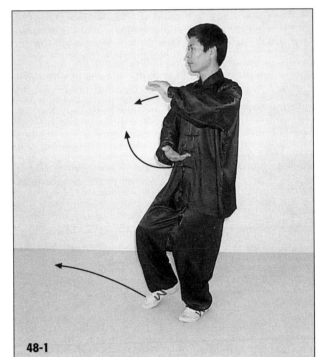

48-1

Posture 48

GRASP BIRD'S TAIL—RIGHT

Movement 1

Shift your weight onto your right leg and turn your body to the right, to 6 o'clock. As you shift your weight away from your left leg, turn your left toes inward to point to 6 o'clock. Move your left arm up and to the right in a curve, while moving your right hand down in a curve. Shift your weight back onto your left leg and bring your right foot next to your left, toes touching the floor. At the same time, move your left hand down in front of your chest, with the palm facing down, and turn your right palm face up at abdomen level to form a hold-ball position with your left hand. Look at your left hand.

163

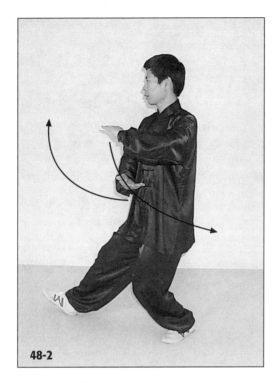

48-2

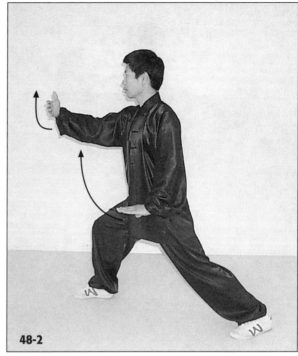

48-2

Movement 2

Turn your body slightly to the right and step your right foot to 10 o'clock. Continue turning your body to the right to 9 o'clock and shift your weight onto your right leg to form a right bow stance. Move your right forearm up to shoulder level, with your palm facing inward and your elbow bending as if warding off a coming attack, while dropping your left hand slowly to the side of your left hip, with the palm facing down. Look at your right forearm.

☑ Key Points

1. Make sure your right heel touches the floor first when taking the right step. As your body weight shifts forward, press down your right sole to make your whole right foot touch the floor.

2. Keep both arms rounded. Keep your shoulders and elbows sunk.

3. Coordinate your hands' separation with the turning of your body and the bending of your right leg.

4. Keep a 12-inch transverse distance between your feet when forming the bow stance.

5. Face 9 o'clock in the final position.

☑ Self-Defense Application

This is called the "Ward Off" movement. Use your right forearm to intercept your attacker's hand and dissolve the force by turning your body to the right. Bring your left arm down and pluck your hand to protect yourself from the attacker's kick.

Grasp Bird's Tail is composed of four techniques: ward off, roll back, press and push. They are linked together to deflect an attack, and to pull or push an attacker off balance.

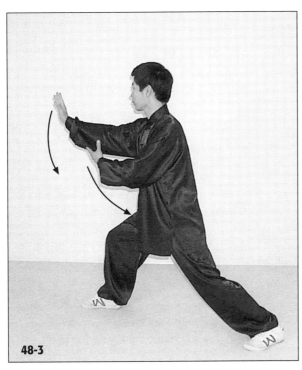

48-3

Movement 3

Turn your body slightly to the right, to a position between 9 and 10 o'clock, and extend your right hand forward, with the palm turning down as if grabbing something. Turn your left palm up and forward, and bring your left hand up across your abdomen until it is just below your right forearm. Then, turn your body slowly to the left, to 7 o'clock, and shift your weight back to your left leg. At the same time, pull both hands back, down, up, and to the left, in a curve, until your left hand is at shoulder level with the palm facing up, and your right hand is in front of your chest with the palm facing inward. Your eyes should follow your left hand.

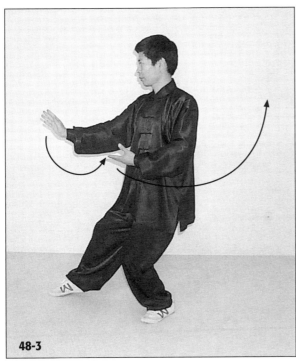

48-3

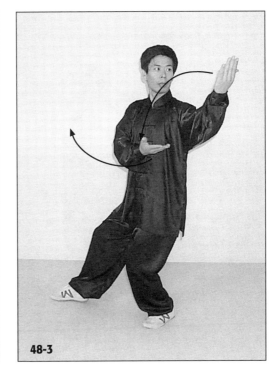

48-3

☑ Key Points

1. Pull back both arms in a circular movement as your body turns and your weight shifts back.

2. Keep your right foot flat on the floor. Do not lean your body forward or protrude your buttocks. Maintain your body in the center and root your feet into the ground to keep them solid and your body flexible.

3. Face 7 o'clock in the final position.

☑ Self-Defense Application

This is called a "Roll Back" movement. It allows you to hold your attacker's elbow and wrist to destroy balance. The pulling is energized through turning your waist and shifting your body weight backward.

Movement 4

Turn your body slowly to the right, to 9 o'clock. Bend your left arm and bring your left hand to the inside of your right wrist. Shift your body weight to your right leg into a right bow stance while pressing both hands forward with your right palm facing inward and your left palm facing outward. Look at your right wrist.

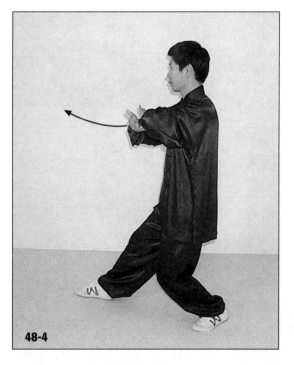

48-4

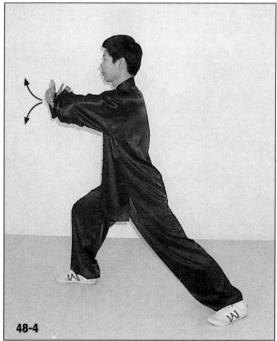

48-4

☑ Key Points

1. Pressing your hands forward must be coordinated with your body turning and your weight shifting forward. The pressing force comes from your waist and spine, in addition to your body weight. Press with a continuous pressure.

2. Keep both arms rounded and relaxed. Keep a 1-inch distance between your palms. Keep both shoulders sunk.

3. Keep your body erect. Do not lean forward when your hands press out. Keep both feet flat on the floor.

4. Face 9 o'clock in the final position.

☑ Self-Defense Application

This is called the "Press Out" movement. Use the flow of your body weight to press your right hand and forearm against your attacker's chest.

Movement 5

Following the press out motion, separate your hands to a shoulder-width and turn both palms forward and down. Sit back and shift your weight onto your left leg, raising up your right toes. At the same time, draw both hands back and down in a curve to the front of your abdomen, with the palms pressing down. Transfer your body weight slowly onto your right leg, while

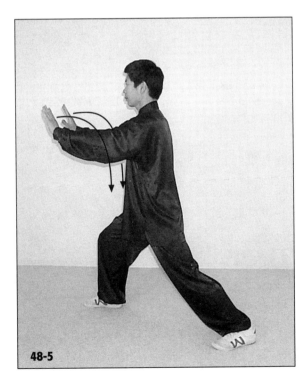

48-5

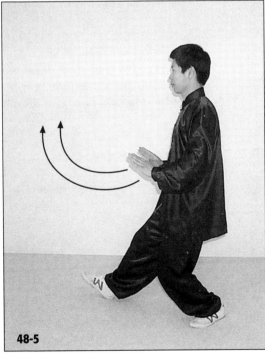

48-5

pushing both palms forward and upward in a curve to shoulder level. Bend your right knee to form a right bow stance. Look to the front.

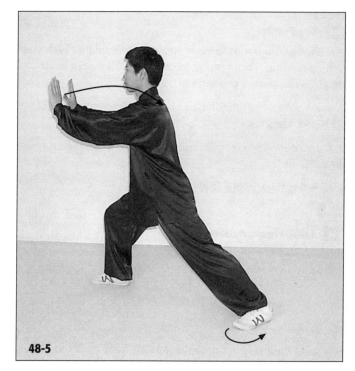

48-5

 Key Points

1. Keep your waist and hips relaxed. Do not shrug your shoulder when pushing out your hands. Keep the elbows slightly down.

2. Coordinate your hands pushing with your body shifting forward. Use your body to generate the push instead of your arms.

3. Do not push your body weight too far forward. Your right knee should be behind your right toes.

4. Face 9 o'clock in the final position.

 Self-Defense Application

This is called the "Push Out" movement. Sit back and draw your hands back to protect yourself and avoid an attack. Then, pin your attacker's arms down and push toward his chest. Push upward and forward to destroy the attacker's balance.

Posture 49

CROSS HANDS

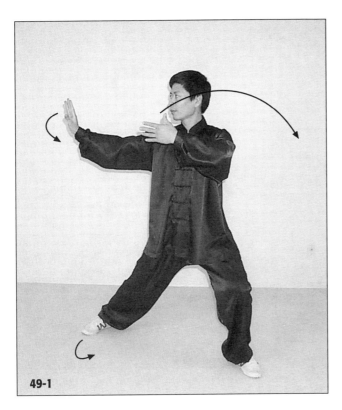

49-1

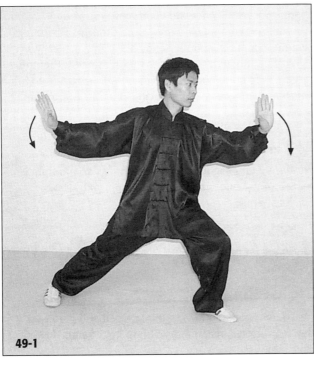

49-1

Movement 1

Rotate your left toes toward 6 o'clock, as you sit back and shift your body weight onto your left leg. Turn your body to the left, to 5 o'clock, with your right toes turning toward 6 o'clock. At the same time, move your left hand in a horizontal curve at the shoulder level to your left side with the left palm turning slowly outward and downward. Look at your left hand.

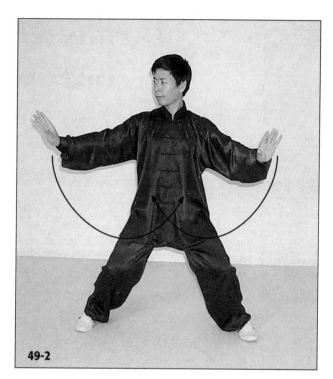

49-2

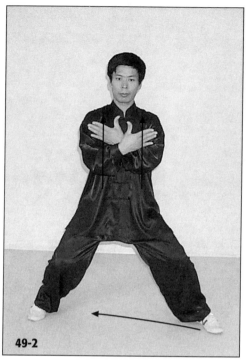

49-2

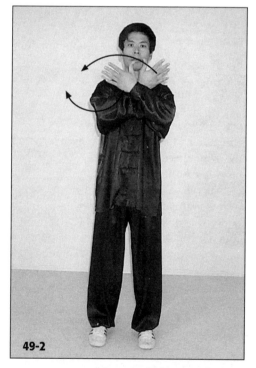

49-2

Movement 2

Shift your body weight slowly onto your right leg and bring your left foot toward your right foot, so they are parallel and a shoulder-width apart. Straighten both legs gradually and move both hands down in a vertical curve to cross at the wrist in front of your abdomen. Then move your hands up to shoulder level with your right hand nearer to your body, palms facing inward. Look to the front.

☑ Key Points

1. Place your weight evenly on both legs as your hands cross. Keep both arms in an arc shape, with elbows slightly bent.

2. Keep your body erect as you straighten your legs.

3. Face 6 o'clock in the final position.

☑ Self-Defense Application

As you sit back and turn to the left, pull and grab your left hand to deflect an attack. Bring both hands down in a circular motion and then up to protect your front body.

End of Sequence 3

It is optional to stop here, closing the form with Posture 74 (see page 226), or you can continue to practice with Sequence 4.

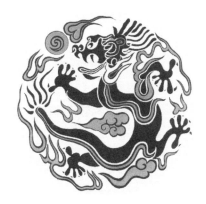

Sequence 4

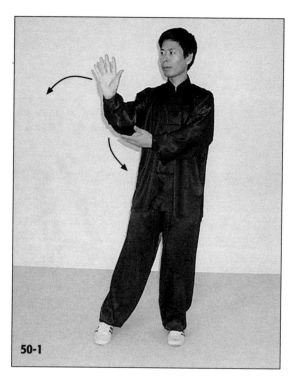

50-1

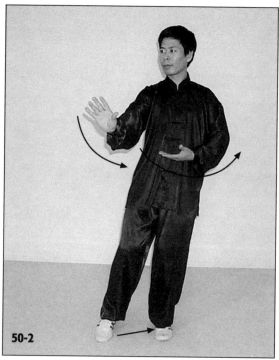

50-2

Posture 50

ROLL BACK AND PRESS OUT—RIGHT

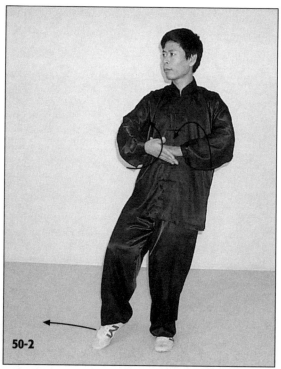

50-2

Movement 1

Shift your weight onto your right leg and rotate your left toes inward slightly. Then, turn your body to the right, to a position between 7 and 8 o'clock. Drop your left palm under your right forearm, palm facing up. Turn the right palm facing out. Look at your right hand.

Movement 2

Shift your weight back onto your left leg and raise up your right heel, toes touching the floor. At the same time, move your right hand forward and your left hand back toward your chest. Without any pause, turn your body to the left slightly, to 7 o'clock, and roll both arms back and down in a curve to the left side of your waist.

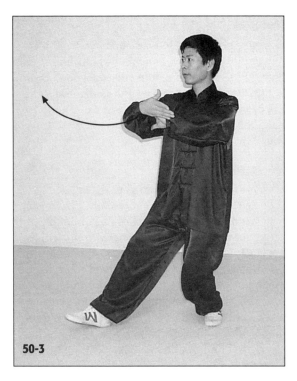

50-3

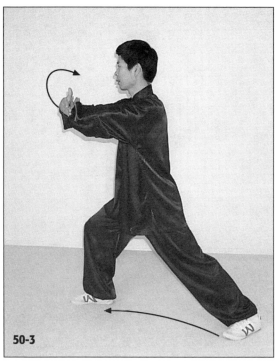

50-3

Bring your right foot back to rest next to your left foot with the toes touching the floor.

Movement 3

Turn your body to the right to 9 o'clock, and step your right foot toward 10 o'clock. Bring both hands up in circular motion and curve your right forearm in front of your chest, with the palm facing inward, while placing your left palm inside of your right wrist. Shift your weight forward onto your right leg to form a right bow stance and press out your right forearm. Look at both hands.

☑ Key Points

1. Curve both arms to form a circle. Your left hand should support your right forearm pressing out.

2. Coordinate right hands pressing out with your body shifting forward.

3. Face 9 o'clock in the final position.

☑ Self-Defense Application

Extend your right hand to grab an attacker's arm at the elbow and hold the wrist with your left hand to pull to your rear left. Turn your right forearm against the chest with the support of your left hand. Press your attacker by shifting your weight forward.

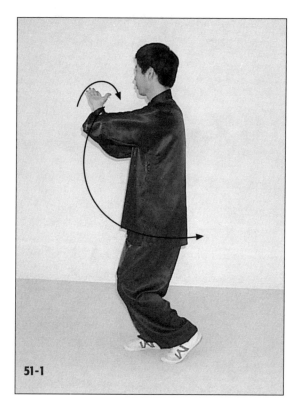

51-1

Posture 51

BRUSH KNEE AND PUNCH DOWN

Movement 1

As your weight shifts forward, bring your left foot forward just behind your right, toes touching the floor. At the same time, turn your right hand in an outward and upward curve to shoulder level, with the palm facing up. Keep the fingers of your left hand touching the inside of your right wrist. Look at your right hand.

Movement 2

Shift your weight back onto your left leg and lift your right heel off the floor. Continue to turn your right hand clockwise in a flat circle in front of your right shoulder. Turn your body to the left, to 7 o'clock, and lower your left hand to your left side. Then, bring your left hand up in a circular motion to your rear left at ear level, and move your right hand down and to the left in a curve to waist level. Step your right foot toward 10 o'clock, heel touching the floor.

Movement 3

Turn your body to the right to 9 o'clock and shift your weight forward onto your right leg to form a right bow stance. At the same time, brush your right hand to the outside of your right knee, palm facing down. Clench your left hand into a fist to punch down and forward in front of your body at waist level, with the back of your fist facing outward. Look diagonally downward.

Key Points

1. Keep your waist and hips relaxed and your upper body erect.

2. Do not lean your left shoulder down as you punch down with your left fist.

3. Turning your right palm in a flat circle is a popular hand motion in the Wu style. Turn your waist in the same circle pattern as your palm.

4. This posture combines the motion of the Wu-style hand and Sun-style step.

5. Face 9 o'clock in the final position.

Self-Defense Application

Turn your right palm to deflect an attacker's hand and move closer. Continue to block off the arm with your right hand circling down and to the left. Punch your left fist into your attacker's lower abdomen.

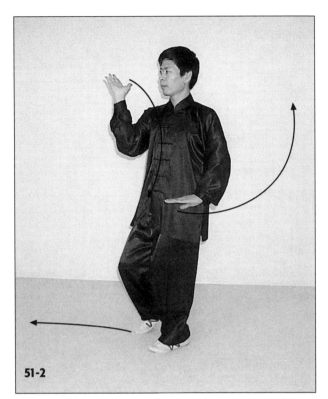

51-2

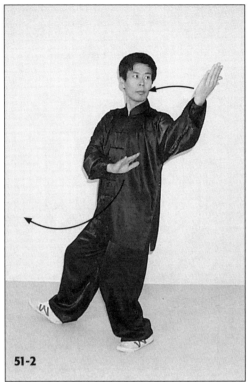

51-2

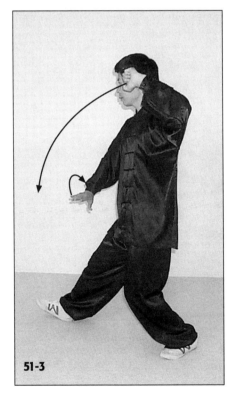

51-3

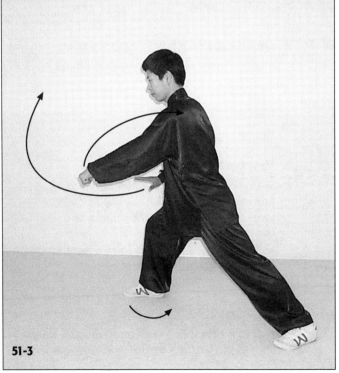

51-3

177

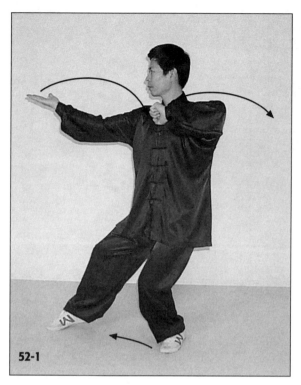

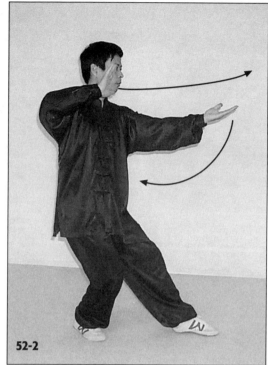

Posture 52

WHITE SNAKE FLICKS ITS TONGUE

Movement 1

Shift your weight onto your left leg and turn your body to the left slightly. At the same time, move your right palm up to shoulder level and pull your left fist up and in a curve to the left in front of your chest. Look at your right palm.

Movement 2

Turn your right toes inward and shift your weight back to your right leg. Continue to turn your body to the left, to 3 o'clock, and turn your left toes outward to 2 o'clock. At the same time,

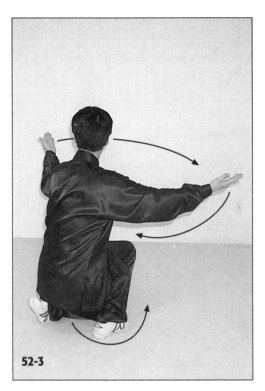

52-3

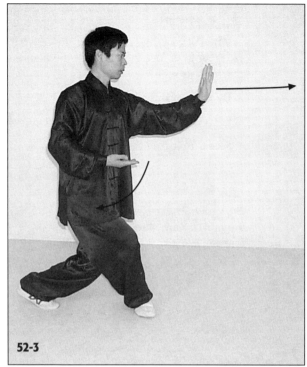

52-3

open your left fist and pull it down and back to the left side of your waist, while pushing your right palm out at shoulder level. Squat down half way into a resting stance, with your left leg in front, crossing over your right knee. Look at your right hand.

Movement 3

Move your left hand in a curve to your rear left side at shoulder level, with the palm rotating up. Turn your right palm up. Stand up slightly and step your right foot in front of your left foot, then squat down into another resting stance with your right leg crossing over your left knee. At the same time, push your left palm out at shoulder level and pull your right palm back to the right side of your waist. Look at your left hand.

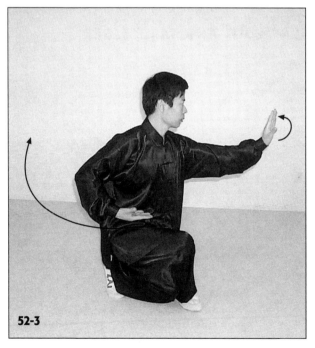

52-3

☑ Key Points

1. When you assume the resting stance, your back leg's knee should be behind your front leg's calf. Your front foot should touch the floor entirely, but your back foot should touch the floor only with its toes.

2. Do not straighten your arm while pushing forward. Keep it flexible.

3. Keep your body erect. Do not lean forward as you push out your palm.

4. Face 3 o'clock in the final position.

☑ Self-Defense Application

Grab your attacker's wrist with your left hand and put your right hand under the armpit to lift the body up and throw it over your rear left. Then, alternate pushing your left and right palms forward, like a snake flicking its tongue.

Posture 53

SLAP FOOT AND TAME TIGER

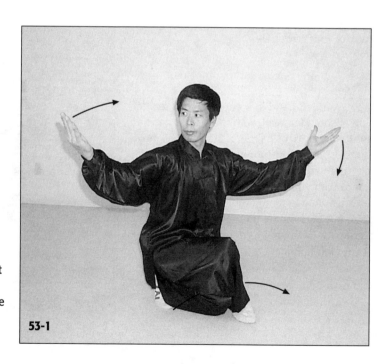

53-1

Movement 1

Stand up and step your left foot forward, toes turning outward. At the same time, turn your left palm face up and curve your right hand up to the rear right at shoulder level. Look to the front.

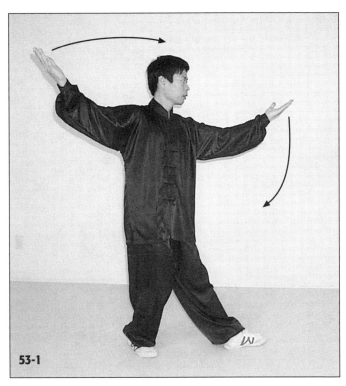

53-1

Movement 2

Shift your weight onto your left leg and kick your right foot up in front of your body, with the instep flat. Slap it with your right palm. At the same time, move your left palm down, then up to your rear left at ear level.

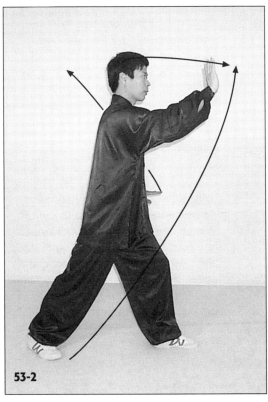

53-2

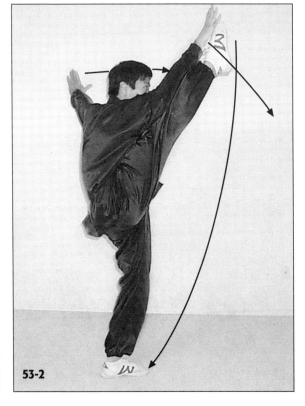

53-2

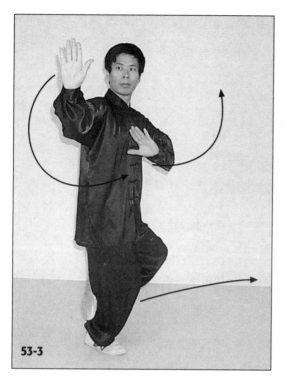

53-3

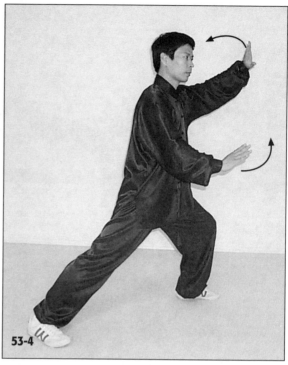

53-4

53-4

Movement 3

Cross your right foot down to the left side of your left foot and shift your weight onto it, while lifting your left foot. At the same time, rotate and swing both arms clockwise to the right as you turn your body to the right, to 4 o'clock. Look at your right hand.

Movement 4

Step your left foot toward 2 o'clock and shift your weight onto it to form a bow stance. Continue to swing both hands clockwise across your waist to the left side of your body. Clench both hands into fists. Move your left fist up to head level with the fist eye facing obliquely down, and move your right fist next to your left ribs with the fist eye facing inward. Look at your right side.

☑ Key Points

1. Keep your left leg bent slightly when you kick your right foot up. Keep a firm standing position as you kick.

2. Kick your right foot as high as you can with the toes straight up. Step your right foot down lightly and gently.

3. Keep both arms in an arc shape in the final position. Relax your chest, hips, and waist.

4. Face 4 o'clock in the final position.

☑ Self-Defense Application

Step your left leg forward, closer to your attacker, and kick your right foot at the chin or neck. Step to the left to avoid a return attack, while circling both arms in front of your body to protect yourself. Then, punch your left fist toward the head, and punch your right fist to the ribs.

Posture 54

THROW FIST DIAGONALLY ASIDE–RIGHT

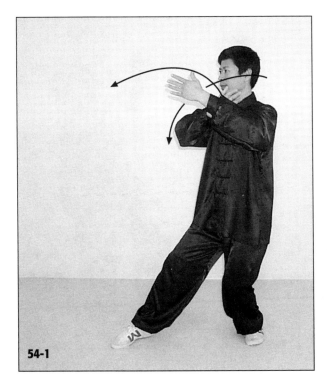

54-1

Movement 1

Shift your weight onto your right leg and turn your left toes inward while turning your body to the right, to 6 o'clock. At the same time, open both fists and move your left forearm to the right, with your palm turning upward. Move your right palm up to just inside your left forearm. Look at your left hand.

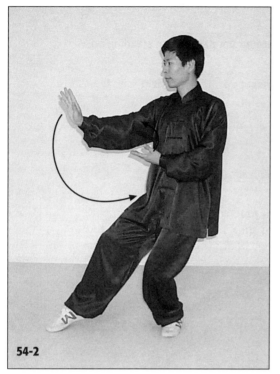

54-2

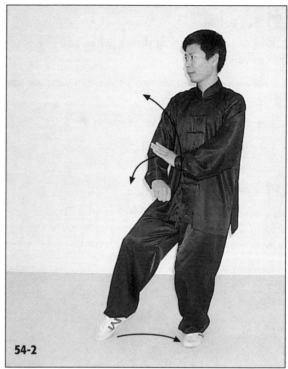

54-2

Movement 2

Shift your weight back to your left leg and continue turning your body to the right, to 8 o'clock. Meanwhile, extend your right hand over your left forearm, as if to catch something, while moving your left hand down under your right elbow. Circle both arms clockwise to the left and bring your right foot back next to your left foot, with the toes touching the floor. Clench your right hand into a fist as you pull it toward your abdomen and move your left hand inside your right forearm. Look at a 9 o'clock position.

Movement 3

Step your right foot toward 10 o'clock and shift your weight onto your right leg to form a right bow stance. At the same time, circle your right hand up and forward, punching your right fist

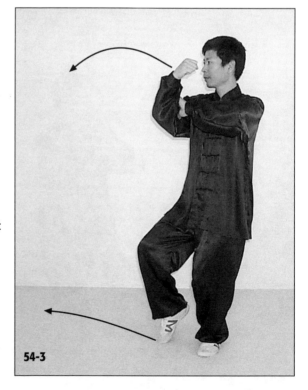

54-3

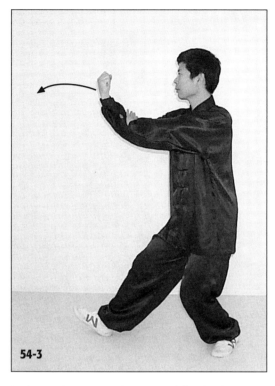

54-3

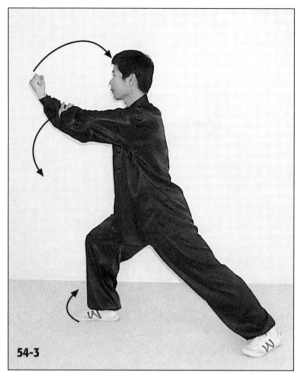

54-3

in front of you with the back of the fist facing outward, while placing your left palm on top of your right forearm to enforce the punch. Look at your right fist.

☑ Key Points

1. Twist and circle your waist to lead your arms in a circular motion.

2. Keep your waist and shoulders relaxed when you throw out your right fist.

3. Do not lean your upper body forward when you punch.

4. Turn about 180 degrees from the left to the right.

5. Face 9 o'clock in the final position.

☑ Self-Defense Application

Turn and block your right side with your left forearm. Grab your attacker's arm with your right hand and pull toward you. Circle your right hand back and into a fist to punch your attacker's chest, with your left hand touching your right forearm to enforce the hit.

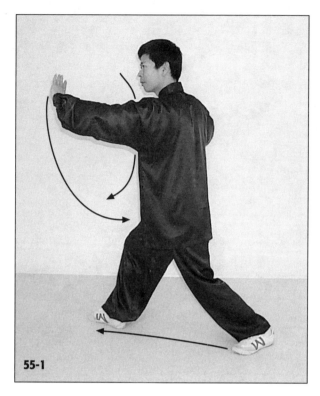

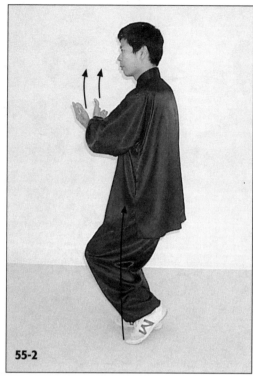

55-1

55-2

Posture 55

KICK WITH LEFT TOES

Movement 1

Sit back to shift your weight onto your left leg and separate your hands, with your right fist opening. Raise your right toes and turn them outward slightly.

Movement 2

Shift your weight forward to your right leg and bring your left foot up near your right, toes touching the floor. At the same time, bring both palms down in a circular motion in front of your abdomen, with your hands crossing each other. Your left hand should be on the bottom and both palms should be face up.

Movement 3

Lift your left leg while holding both hands up in front of your chest. Kick your left foot out toward 9 o'clock, with the toes pointing forward. At the same time, separate your hands and extend your left hand out just above your kicking leg, palm facing forward. Extend your right hand to your rear right at shoulder level, with the palm facing outward. Look at your left foot.

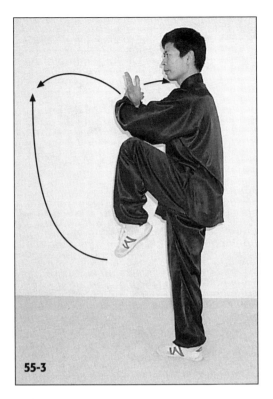

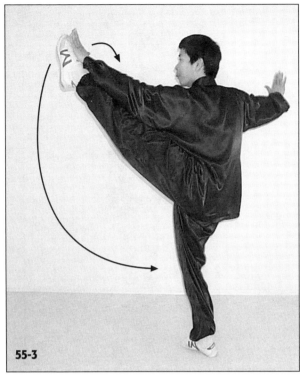

55-3

55-3

✔ Key Points

1. Keep your standing leg bent slightly to hold a good balance.

2. Keep your upper body naturally upright. Do not lean forward.

3. Keep both arms bent at the elbows and circle your arms smoothly in front of your body.

4. Face 9 o'clock in the final position.

✔ Self-Defense Application

Separate your hands to block your attacker's arms and raise your left foot to kick at the head or abdomen. Extend your left arm above your left leg to protect against being grabbed.

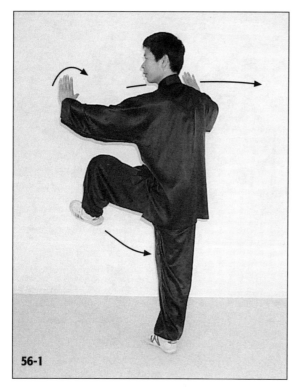

56-1

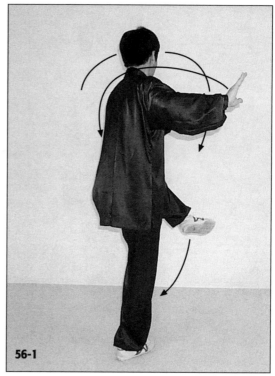

56-1

Posture 56

TURN TO KICK WITH RIGHT TOES

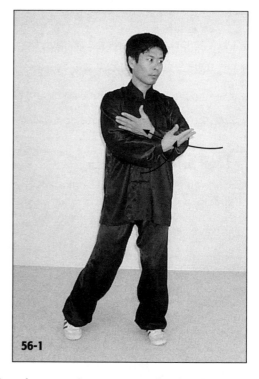

56-1

Movement 1

Draw your left leg back by bending it at the knee and turn your body 270 degrees to the right, to 6 o'clock, balancing on your right toes. Step your left foot down next to your right foot, and shift your weight onto your left leg. Keep your right toes touching the floor. Move your hands down and around in a curve to cross each other in front of your abdomen, with your right hand on the bottom.

Movement 2

Lift your right leg while holding both hands up in front of your chest. Kick your right foot out toward 9 o'clock, with the toes pointing forward. At the same time, separate your hands and

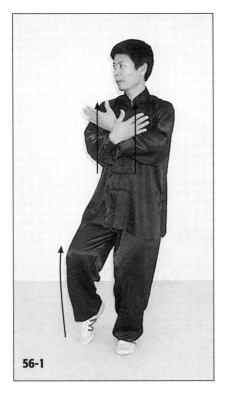

56-1

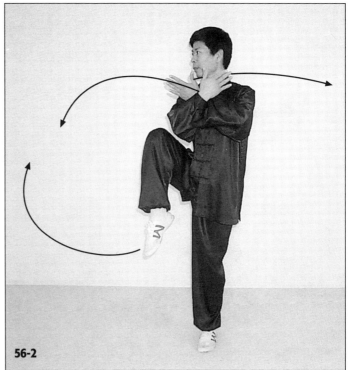

56-2

extend your right hand out just above your kicking leg, palm facing forward. Extend your left hand to your rear left at shoulder level, with the palm facing outward. Look at your right foot.

☑ Key Points

1. Keep your standing leg bent slightly to hold a good balance.

2. Keep your upper body naturally upright. Do not lean forward.

3. Keep both arms bent at the elbows and circle your arms smoothly in front of your body.

4. Face 9 o'clock in the final position.

☑ Self-Defense Application

Separate your hands to block your attacker's arms and raise your right foot to kick at the head or abdomen.

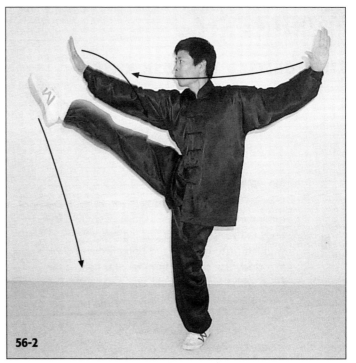

56-2

Extend your right arm above your right leg to protect against being grabbed.

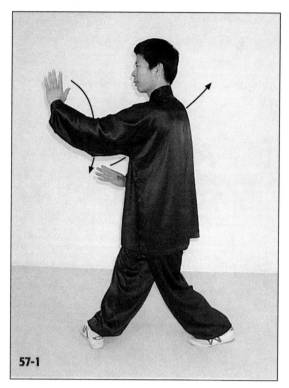

57-1

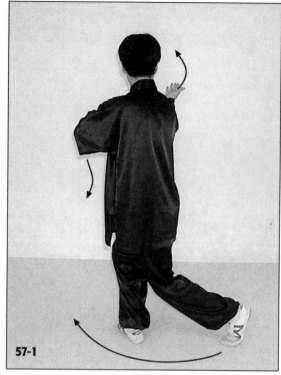

57-1

Posture 57

STEP FORWARD TO BRUSH KNEE AND PUSH PALM

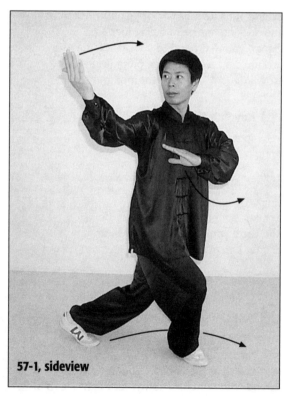

57-1, sideview

Movement 1

Step your right foot down with the toes turning outward to 10 o'clock. Turn your body to the right, to 9 o'clock. Move your left hand forward and bring it down in a clockwise circle in front of your right chest with the palm facing down while moving your right hand back toward your chest. Bring your right hand down, in a circular motion, and then up counterclockwise to your rear right at shoulder level, with the palm rotating upward. Look at your right palm.

190

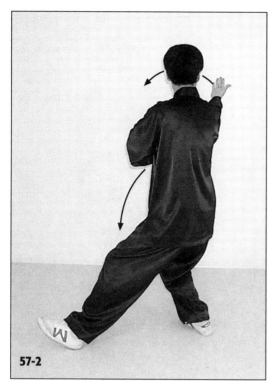

57-2

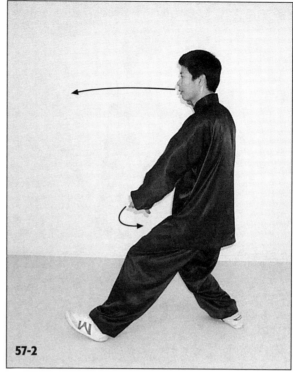

57-2

Movement 2

Step your left foot forward toward 8 o'clock and shift your weight onto your left leg to form a left bow stance. At the same time, bend your right arm at the elbow and push your right palm forward, toward 9 o'clock, passing your right ear, while moving your left hand down across your abdomen to the left side of your left knee. Look at your right hand.

 Key Points

1. Synchronize pushing your right hand out with shifting your weight forward.

2. Sink your shoulders and drop your elbow when you push your right hand out.

3. Do not lean your body forward. Keep your waist and hips relaxed.

4. Face 9 o'clock in the final position.

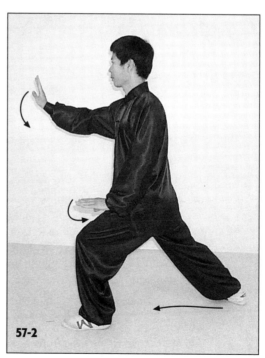

57-2

 Self-Defense Application

Both hands take turns circling and blocking in front of your body. Step toward your attacker and push the upper body with your right hand.

191

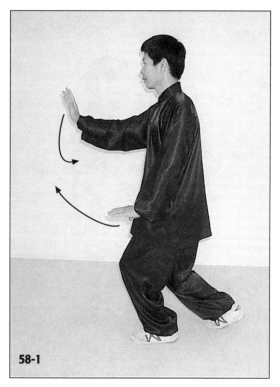

58-1

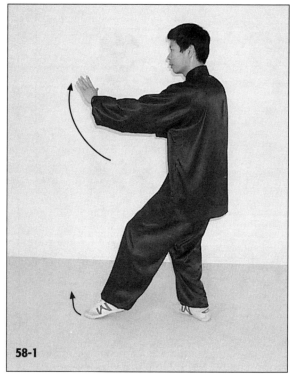

58-1

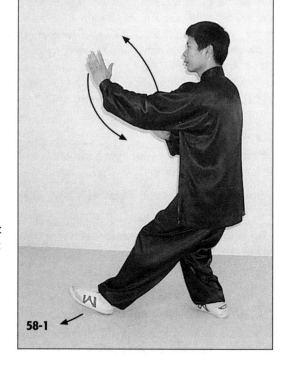

58-1

Posture 58

PLAY GUITAR–LEFT

Bring your right foot forward next to your left heel, then shift your weight onto your right leg. Raise your left foot and take a small step forward to form a left empty stance with your heel touching the floor. At the same time, raise your left hand in front of your body to nose level with your arm slightly bent and your palm facing right, while moving your right hand to the left and then down to the inside of your left elbow, palm facing left. Look at your left fingertips. Face 9 o'clock.

☑ Key Points

1. Hold your shoulders and elbows down. Coordinate your arms' motion with your waist turning.

2. Keep your body erect and natural, your chest relaxed. Bend both knees slightly in the empty stance.

3. Face 6 o'clock in the final position.

☑ Self-Defense Application

Intercept and grab an attacker's wrist using your right hand. Move your left palm up to hold and press the elbow against your right hand. Squeeze both palms in to bend an attacker's elbow.

Posture 59

FAIR LADY WORKS WITH SHUTTLE

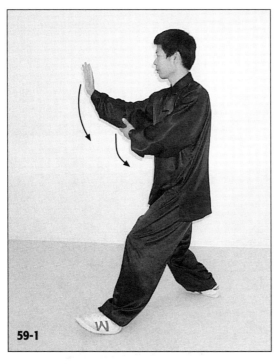

59-1

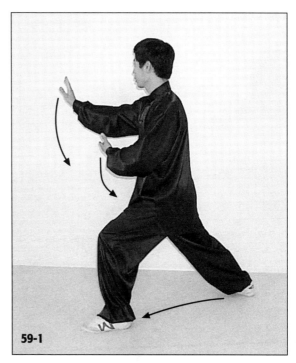

59-1

Movement 1

Move your left foot to the left slightly and shift your weight onto your left leg to form a left bow stance. Face 10 o'clock. At the same time, extend your right palm to the right, crossing over your left hand, while turning your left palm up and circling it to the right and then back under your right elbow. Both hands should move in a clockwise arc. Look at your right hand.

Movement 2

Shift all your weight onto your left leg and turn your body to the left, to 8 o'clock. At the same time, roll both hands back and to the left in a downward curve, while bringing your right foot next to your left, toes touching the floor. Your eyes should follow your right hand.

Movement 3

Continue circling both hands up to chest level, with your right palm rotating inward. Place your left palm on your right wrist. Step your right foot toward 10 o'clock and shift your weight onto your right leg to form a right bow stance. Press your right forearm forward. Look at your hands.

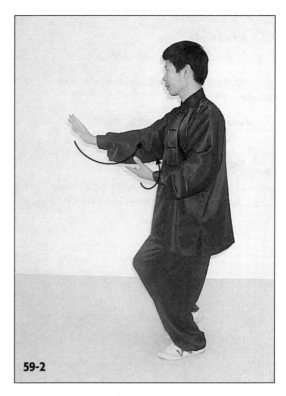

59-2

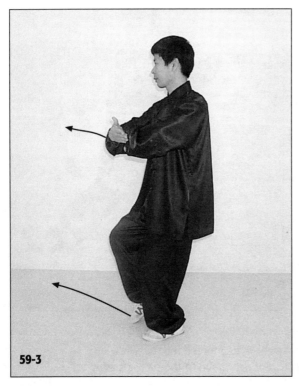

59-3

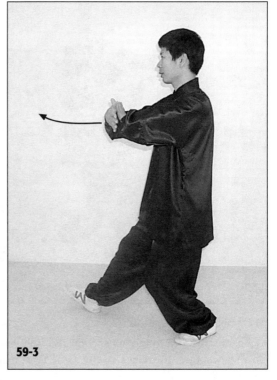

59-3

194

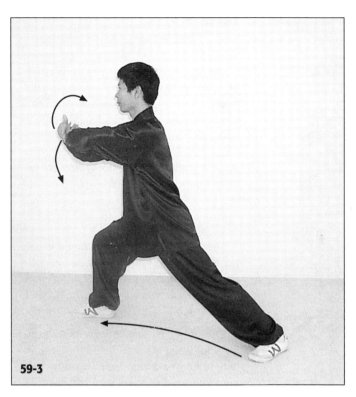

59-3

Movement 4

Without any pause, shift your weight onto your right leg and bring your left foot next to your right, toes touching the floor. At the same time, rotate your right hand in a flat clockwise circle to the right. Shift your weight back to your left leg and lift your right heel, your toes still touching the floor, while completing the flat circle with your right palm and moving your left hand closer to your left ribs.

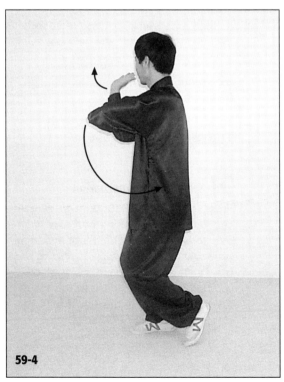

59-4

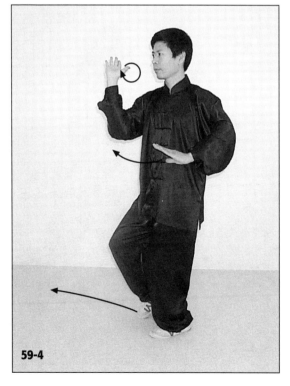

59-4

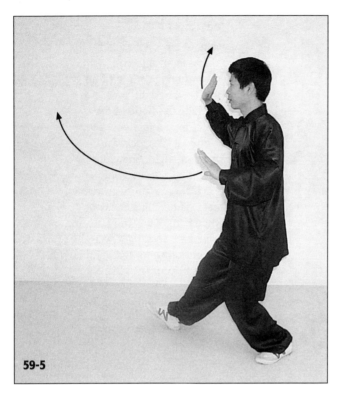

59-5

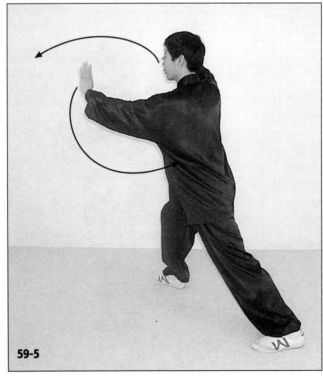

59-5

Movement 5

Step your right foot toward a position between 10 and 11 o'clock and shift your weight onto your right leg to form a right bow stance. Turn your right palm to face forward and raise your right forearm to the right side of your head, while pushing your left hand toward a position between 10 and 11 o'clock. Look to the front. The arrows in the bottom photograph show transition to Posture 60.

☑ Key Points

1. There are three styles combined in this posture. It starts with a Wu-style flat hand circle, continues with a Sun-style follow-up half step, and finishes with a Yang-style Fair Lady push.

2. Coordinate circling your palm with twisting your waist. Raising your right forearm should be coordinated with bending your right knee and pushing your left palm forward.

3. Keep a transverse distance of 12 inches between your heels in the bow stance.

4. Do not raise your shoulder when you move your right forearm up to your right forehead.

5. Face a position between 10 and 11 o'clock in the final position.

☑ Self-Defense Application

Press your attacker with your right forearm, your left hand supporting your right wrist. Step forward with your left foot and bring your right foot closer, while deflecting the hand with your right palm and pushing your left hand onto the chest. This follow-up step is popular in the Sun style to get closer to your opponent quickly.

Posture 60

STEP BACK AND SPEAR LEFT PALM

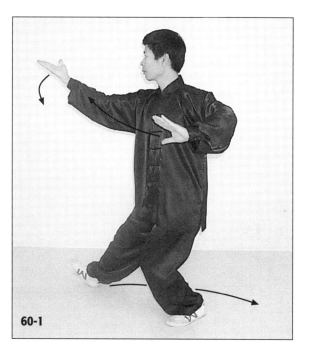

60-1

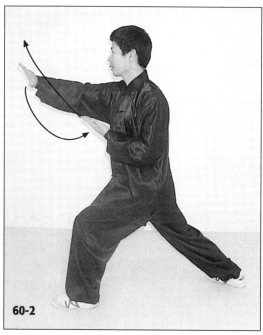

60-2

Movement 1

Shift your weight back to your left leg and turn your body to the left, to 8 o'clock, while raising your right toes. At the same time, move your left hand in a curve to the left and then down to the left side of your waist, with the palm facing down, while moving your right hand to the left and then down in front of your left chest, with the palm facing up. Look at your right palm.

Movement 2

Step your right foot back toward 2 o'clock to form a left bow stance. Pull your right palm back and press it down in front of your left ribs while spearing out your left palm over your right forearm toward 9 o'clock. Rotate your left palm facing up, as you spear it forward; rotate your right palm facing down, as you press it down. Look at your left hand. Arrows in bottom photograph show transition to Posture 61.

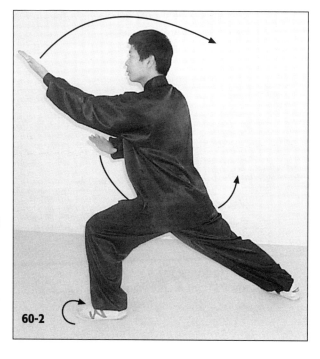

60-2

✅ Key Points

This is a Wu-style posture. Form a bow stance by stepping back, as in Posture 45 (page 156), but with the opposite hands and feet. Face 9 o'clock in the final position.

✅ Self-Defense Application

Step your right leg back to set up a firm bow stance. Lower your right palm to block an attacker's arm. Grab and pull the arm down and thrust your left palm from your waist with your fingers pointing toward your attacker's neck.

Posture 61

PRESS DOWN PALM IN AN EMPTY STANCE

Movement 1

Shift your weight onto your right leg and turn your left toes inward while turning your body to the right about 180 degrees to 3 o'clock. Raise your left hand over your left forehead and press your right hand down in front of your right abdomen.

Movement 2

Shift your weight back to your left leg while raising your right heel, with right toes touching the floor, to form a right empty stance. At the same time, bend

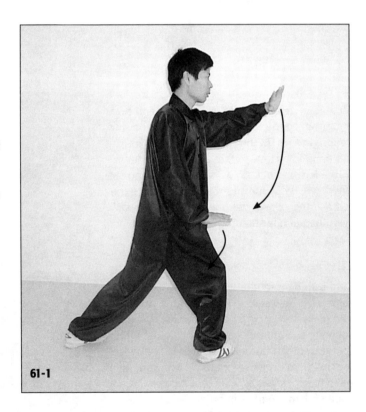

61-1

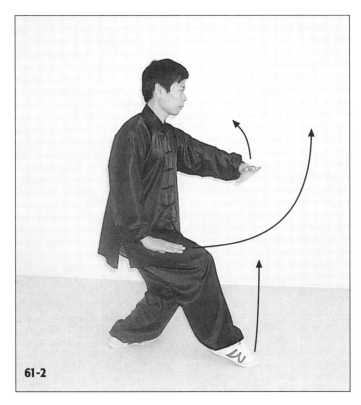

61-2

both knees to lower your body and press your left palm down above your right knee with the fingers pointing to the right. Your right palm should be held down at the side of your right hip. Look at your left hand.

☑ Key Points

1. This posture comes from the Sun style. It emphasizes the left forearm pressing down.

2. The pressing motion is driven by lowering your body. Do not lower your left forearm only.

3. Do not bend your body forward when you press your left palm down.

4. Keep your waist and hips relaxed for a smooth 180-degree turn.

5. Face 3 o'clock in the final position.

☑ Self-Defense Application

To protect yourself from an attack from the back, turn around and block down your left forearm vertically in front of your body. Meanwhile, protect your abdomen area with your right hand, pulling it down to the right side.

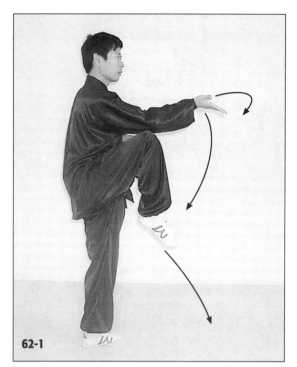

62-1

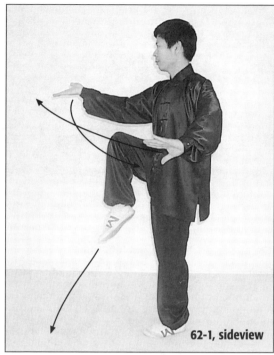

62-1, sideview

Posture 62

STAND ON ONE LEG AND LIFT PALM

Stand on your left leg and lift your right, with the knee fully bent and toes pointing downward. At the same time, turn your body slightly to the left and lift your right palm in front of you to chest level with the palm turning up, while moving your left hand up and to the left to press out at shoulder level, with the palm facing outward. Look at your right hand.

☑ Key Points

1. This posture originated from the Chen style.

2. Lifting your right palm should be coordinated with straightening your left leg.

3. Your right elbow should be just above your right knee.

4. Relax your chest and waist. Keep your shoulders sunk and elbows dropped.

5. Face 3 o'clock in the final position.

☑ Self-Defense Application

Move your left hand in a curve to pull aside an attacker's right arm while lifting up the left arm with your right palm. By controlling both of your attacker's arms, you can kick with your raised right foot.

Posture 63

BUMP WITH LEFT FOREARM IN A HALF HORSE-RIDING STANCE

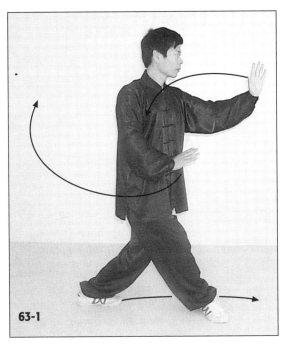

63-1

Movement 1

Step down your right foot in front of you at 4 o'clock, with the toes turning to the right. Shift your weight onto your right leg. Turn your body to the right, to 4 o'clock, and move your left hand forward, up, and to the right, with the palm facing to the right, while pulling your right hand closer to your body in a circle down and to the right. Look to the front.

Movement 2

Shift your weight totally to your right leg and bring your left foot next to your right, toes touching the floor. At the same time, circle your left hand down in front of your chest with the palm facing down, while circling your right hand up to shoulder level with your palm facing up. Look at your right palm.

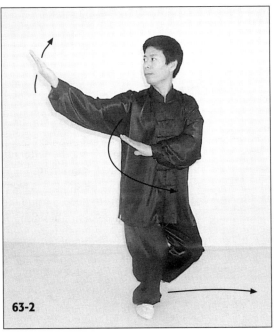

63-2

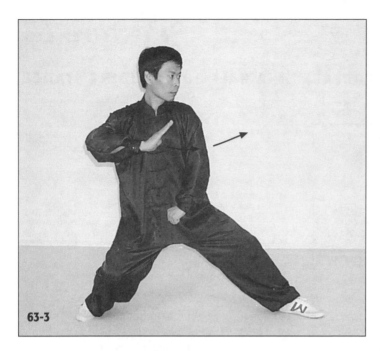

63-3

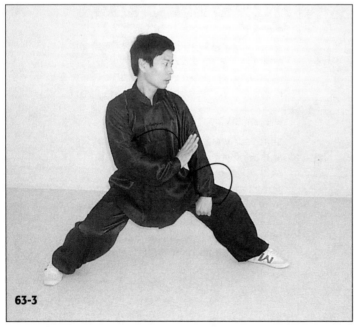

63-3

Movement 3

Step your left foot forward to 3 o'clock, with your left heel touching the floor first. Shift your weight forward slightly to form a half horse-riding stance. Clench your left hand into a fist and continue to circle it down inside your left knee, with the back of the fist facing right, while placing your right palm on the inside of your left forearm to press and bump it forward. Look to your left.

☑ Key Points

1. This posture is in the Chen style. Step your left foot out, scraping the heel along the floor before the foot is set firm.

2. Keep your upper body erect and hold a firm half horse-riding stance.

3. Bump your left forearm forward in a quick tempo. Make sure the bumping power comes from your rear leg, through your waist, onto your left arm.

4. Your front foot should point to 3 o'clock and your chest should face 6 o'clock in the final position.

☑ Self-Defense Application

Step your right foot toward your attacker and swing your left forearm in a circle in front of your body to block a punch. Step your left foot behind to control your attacker's legs and bump against the body, using your left arm, with your right palm enforcing the bump.

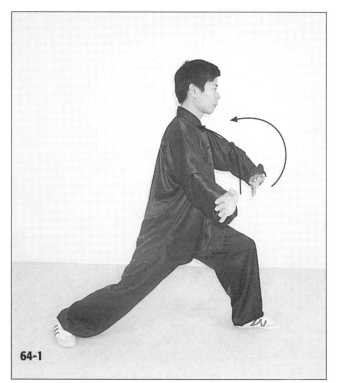

64-1

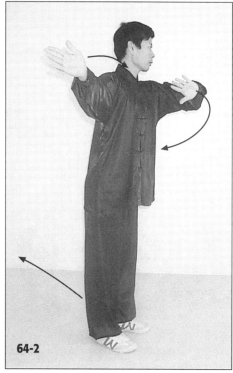

64-2

Posture 64

TURN AROUND WITH LARGE ROLL BACK

Movement 1

Shift your weight onto your right leg and turn your left toes outward. Then shift your weight back to your left leg. Separate your hands and open your left fist into a palm, while rotating both palms to face outward.

Movement 2

Turn your body to the left, to 3 o'clock. Bring your right foot next to your left and stand up. Move both arms up and to the left, your left hand in front of your left shoulder with the palm facing outward and your right hand at the rear right with the palm facing obliquely up. Look to the front.

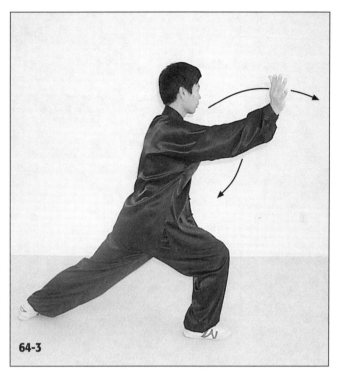

64-3

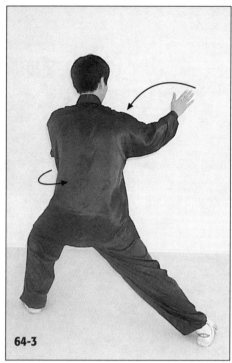

64-3

Movement 3

Shift your weight onto your right leg and step your left foot back to 9 o'clock. Continue to turn your body to the left and pull both arms down and to the left. Look at your right hand.

Movement 4

Turn your body to 12 o'clock. Shift your weight back to your left leg and bend it at the knee, while straightening your right leg and turning your right toes inward. At the same time, move your left hand to the side of your left waist, while lowering your right forearm in front of your chest with both hands clenched into fists. Look at your right fist.

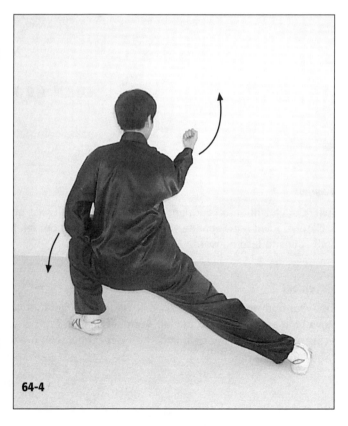

64-4

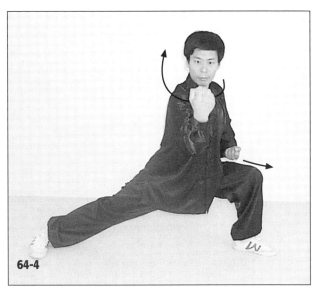

64-4

☑ Key Points

1. Shifting your weight to your left leg should be coordinated with your body turning to the left.

2. The final position looks like a left bow stance, but with the left toes pointing inward slightly. Drop your right elbow and keep an arc shape in your right arm with the fist facing inward. Face 11 o'clock.

☑ Self-Defense Application

Grab your attacker's wrist with your left hand and hold the arm with your right hand. Turn 180 degrees to roll back and pull to your left. Then, rotate your right forearm to press against the elbow.

Posture 65

SCOOP RIGHT PALM

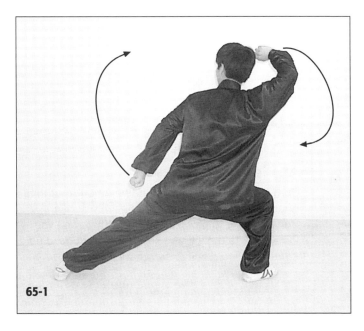

65-1

Movement 1

Shift your weight onto your right leg in a right bow stance and turn your body to the right to 1 o'clock. Move your right forearm in a curve to the upper right quarter of your head with the fist facing obliquely outward, while extending your left hand down and to the left, bringing it to rest above your left thigh with the fist facing obliquely upward. Arrows show transition to Movement 2.

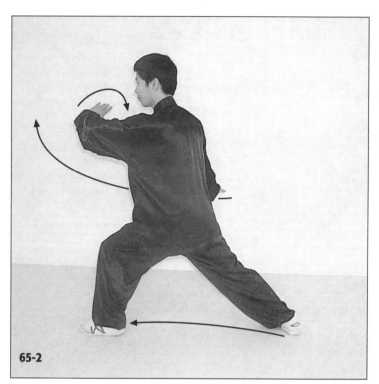

65-2

Movement 2

Turn your left toes outward slightly. Shift your weight onto your left leg and turn your body to the left, to 9 o'clock. Open both fists and move your left hand up and to the right, to the front of your left chest. Move your right hand back and down to the side of your right hip. Look to the front.

Movement 3

Without any pause, bring your right foot next to your left, toes touching the floor, and scoop your right palm up and forward to waist level, while pulling your left palm back to the top of your right forearm. Look at your right palm. Arrows show transition to Posture 66.

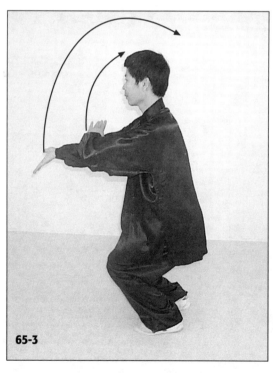

65-3

✔ Key Points

1. Twist your waist to turn your body to the right, then to the left to set up the momentum of scooping your right palm.

2. The T-Stance is a popular position in the Sun style: one leg holds your whole body's weight, with your other toes touching the floor just inside your supporting foot.

3. Keep your shoulders sunk and your upper body erect.

4. Face 9 o'clock in the final position.

✔ Self-Defense Application

Turn your body to the right and bump out your right shoulder and elbow with your right forearm in a curved shape to protect your head. Then, turn your body back to the left and scoop your right hand up to hit your attacker's abdomen area.

Posture 66

SQUAT DOWN TO PENETRATE LEFT PALM

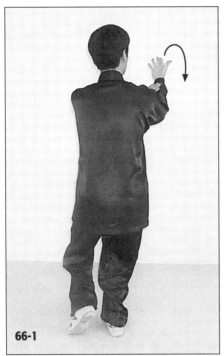

66-1

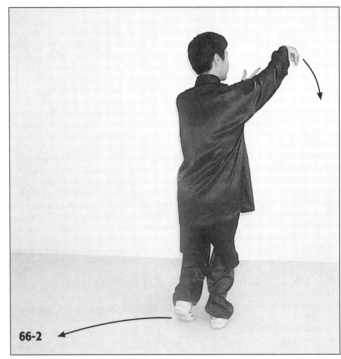

66-2

Movement 1

Turn your body to the right, to 1 o'clock, and drop your right heel, with the whole foot touching the floor, while shifting your weight onto your right leg. At the same time, lift your left heel, leaving the toes touching the floor, while moving both palms up and to the right in a curve, your left palm maintaining contact with your right forearm. Look at your right hand.

Movement 2

Extend your right palm outward. Bunch your fingertips and bend your wrist to form a hook-hand. Step your left foot back and to your left, toward 8 o'clock, toes turning inward. Look at your right hook-hand.

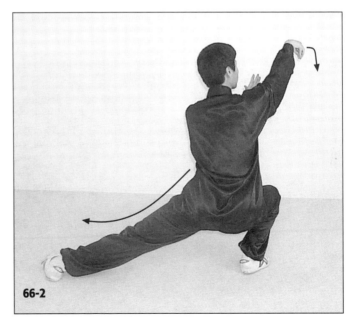

66-2

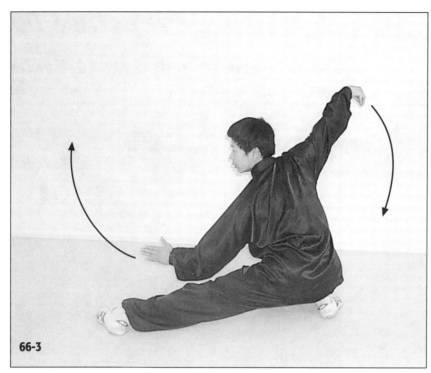

66-3

Movement 3

Squat down and turn your body to the left, to 11 o'clock. Move your left palm down to your left thigh, then slide it forward along the inside of your left leg until it is next to your left foot with the palm facing right. Look at your left hand. Arrows show transition to Posture 67.

☑ Key Points

1. When you squat down, do not let your upper body lean too far forward. Practice lowering your body gradually. Go as low as you can without discomfort.

2. Your bent right knee should point in the same direction as your toes to prevent it from being twisted.

3. Try to stretch your left leg straight out and close to the floor. Keep your left foot fully touching the floor.

4. Face 10 o'clock in the final position.

☑ Self-Defense Application

Squatting down to lower your body is a defensive movement to avoid an attacker's high attack. At the same time, you can extend and stretch your left leg forward and with your left arm under the legs, throw an attacker off balance.

Posture 67

STEP FORWARD AND CROSS FISTS

Movement 1

Turn your left toes slightly out-ward and shift your weight gradually forward onto your left leg to form a left bow stance. Turn your body to the left, to 9 o'clock, and move your left palm up to shoulder level with the palm facing obliquely right-ward, while dropping your right hook-hand behind you with the fingers pointing obliquely upward. Look at your left hand.

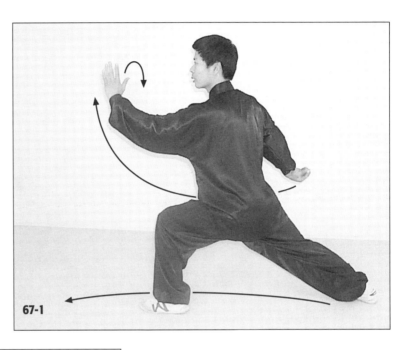

67-1

Movement 2

Step your right foot a small step forward with the toes touching the floor to form a right empty stance. At the same time, clench both hands into fists and move your right fist up and forward to shoulder level, your fists crossing, with your left hand in front of your chest. Your fists should be back to back, with your right fist facing forward and your left fist facing inward. Your right fist should be on the outside. Look at both fists. Arrows show transition to Posture 68.

67-2

☑ Key Points

1. Keep your wrists close to each other and bend both arms at the elbows to form a circle shape.

2. Keep your right leg slightly bent at the knee. Place your weight on your left leg. Keep your hips and waist relaxed.

3. Face 9 o'clock in the final position.

☑ Self-Defense Application

As you shift your weight forward, poke your left hand up to hit an attacker in the lower body. Move your right foot forward into an empty stance and prop up both forearms to fence off an attacker's hands, while kicking with your right foot.

Posture 68

STEP BACK TO RIDE ON TIGER

Movement 1

Step your right foot back to 2 o'clock and turn your body to the right slightly. Open both fists and move your right hand down and to the right in a curve.

Movement 2

Shift your weight onto your right leg and lift your left heel to form a left empty stance. Move your right hand in a circle counterclockwise at the right side of your body, then down to the side of your left thigh with the palm facing obliquely upward, while moving your left hand down and to the left in a curve to the back side of your left hip, palm facing down. Look at your right hand.

Movement 3

Stand on your right leg with your body turning slightly to the left and lift your left

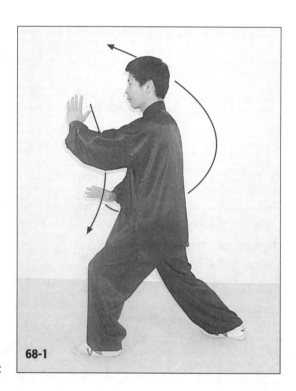

68-1

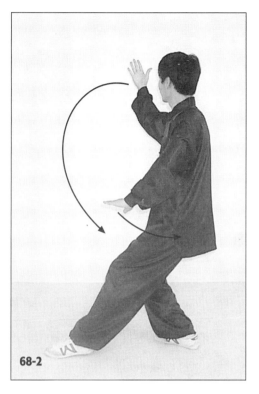

68-2

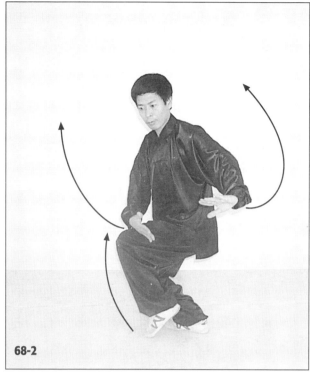

68-2

leg with the knee bent and the toes pointing forward. Keep your left instep flat and turn the sole of your foot toward the right slightly. Move your right hand up and forward in front of you with the palm facing obliquely left, while extending your left hand up to the left to form a hook-hand with the fingers pointing down. Look to the front.

Key Points

1. This posture is popular in the Wu style. Hold your left leg up at a level at which you feel comfortable. Turn your left foot toward the right slightly with the instep flat.

2. Keep your right knee slightly bent to hold a good balance when you stand on your right leg. Keep your body erect.

3. Keep your shoulders sunk and relax your chest.

4. Twist your upper body to the left, to 8 o'clock, in the final position.

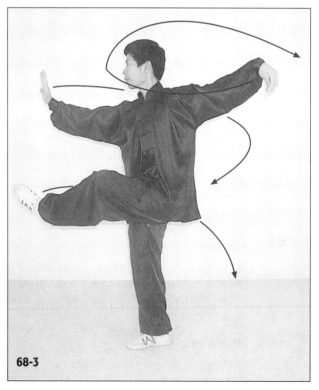

68-3

☑ **Self-Defense Application**

Step back and shift your weight back to avoid an attacker's punch. Circle both arms in front of your body to deflect a hand. After you block down a hand with your right forearm in front of your chest, poke out your right hand in a jerking force toward the chin.

Posture 69

TURN BODY AND SWEEP LOTUS KICK

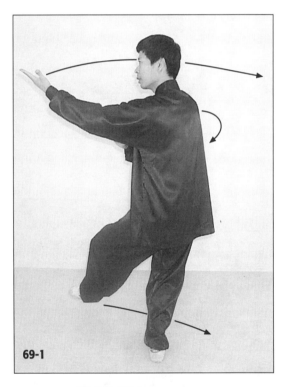

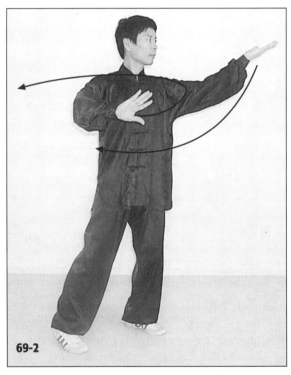

Movement 1

Turn your body to the right, to 2 o'clock, and step your left foot to the right, to 2 o'clock, with the toes turning inward. At the same time, open your left hook-hand and move it all the way to the right, while pulling your right hand back and to the right, to the right side of your body. Look to the front.

Movement 2

Continue to turn your body to the right, to 6 o'clock, and shift your weight to your left leg with toes of your right foot touching the floor. Extend your right hand in a forward curve to the

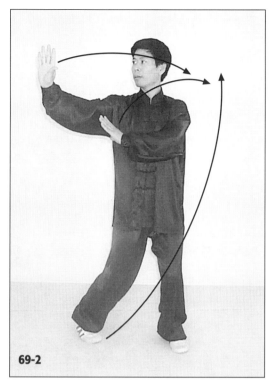

69-2

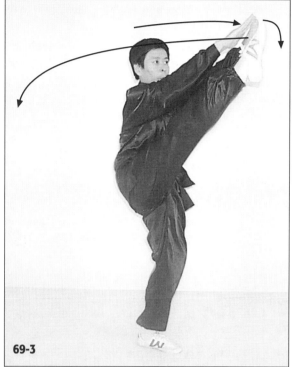

69-3

right, to the right side of your body, with the palm rotating outward to the right. At the same time, pull your left hand down closer to your right ribs with the palm rotating obliquely to the right. Look at your right hand.

Movement 3

Lift your right foot and sweep it in a curve from the upper left, across your face, toward the upper right. Your right leg should be naturally straightened with toes flat. Swing both palms from the right, across your face, and slap the back of your right foot. Look at your hands.

☑ **Key Points**

1. The hand and arm motions of this posture are from Baguazhang, another popular martial arts style.

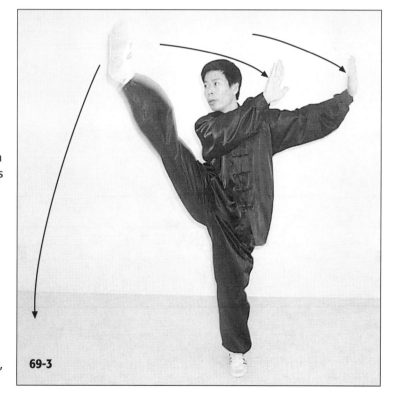

69-3

2. Step your left foot down and pivot on the soles of both feet, turning 270 degrees to the right.

3. Keep your body upright and coordinate your body's turning with your arms moving around your body.

4. Kick your right foot as high as possible. Lean your upper body slightly forward when you sweep with your right foot.

5. Sweep your right foot onto both palms instead of forcing your hands to slap your foot.

6. Face 6 o'clock in the final position.

☑ Self-Defense Application

Turn your body to the right while moving your arms in turn to deflect an attacker's hands. Sweep your right foot, kicking at your attacker's right ear to destroy balance.

Posture 70

PULL BOW TO SHOOT TIGER

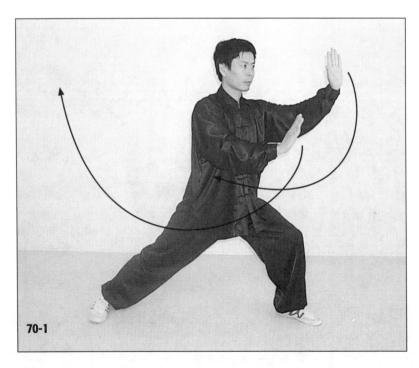

70-1

Movement 1

Drop your right foot at your right side, pointing to 8 o'clock, and extend both palms to the left. Shift your weight onto your right leg and bend it to form a right bow stance. Move both hands down and to the right in a curve with both hands clenched into fists. Bend your left arm at the elbow and place your left fist in front of your right chest.

Movement 2

Turn your body slightly to the left, to 7 o'clock, and punch your left fist forward to 7 o'clock at face level, with the back of the fist facing obliquely inward. At the same time, punch your right fist to the right side of your head at ear level, with the back of the fist facing obliquely inward. Look at your left fist.

☑ Key Points

1. Keep your shoulders sunk and relaxed.

2. Your eyes should follow your hands' movement right, then look at your left fist.

3. After punching out both fists, as if you were bending a bow to shoot something, your left hand should assume a pushing position and your right should assume a pulling position.

4. Face 6 o'clock in the final position.

☑ Self-Defense Application

Swing both arms in front of your body to block an attacker's punch. Punch your left fist forward while curving your right forearm up to protect your head.

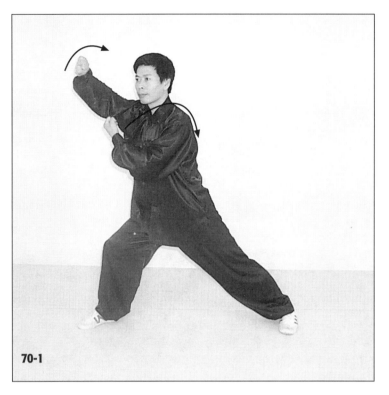

70-1

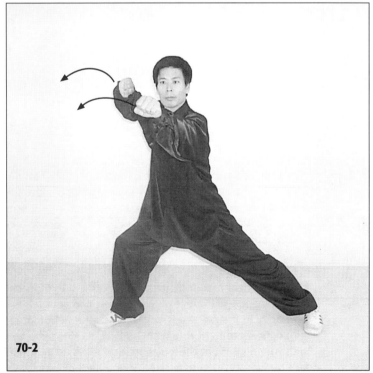

70-2

215

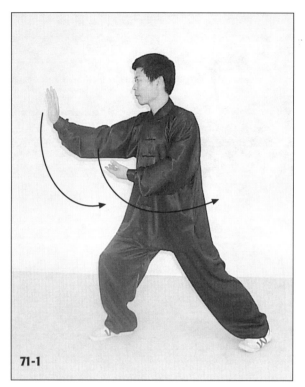

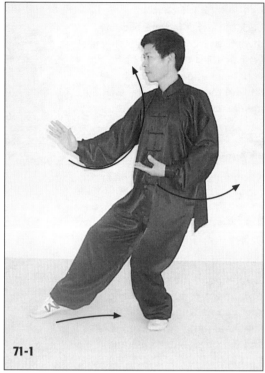

71-1

71-1

Posture 71

HEAD-ON CANNON

Movement 1

Turn your body to the right slightly and open both fists. Move your left hand to the right in front of your chest, while moving your right hand down. Shift your weight back onto your left leg and turn your body to the left, to 6 o'clock. At the same time, rotate both palms to face outward, while moving both hands down and back in a curve to the left. Your eyes should follow your hands.

Movement 2

Move your right foot back, toes touching the floor. Clench both hands into fists, with your right fist moving to the front of your abdomen and your left fist to the left side of your waist. Turn your body to the right, to 8 o'clock, step your right foot forward, and shift your weight onto your right leg to form a right bow stance. At the same time, punch both fists to the front-right, with your right fist at chest level and your left fist at waist level. The backs of both fists should face outward. Concentrate force on the back of your fists. Look at your right fist.

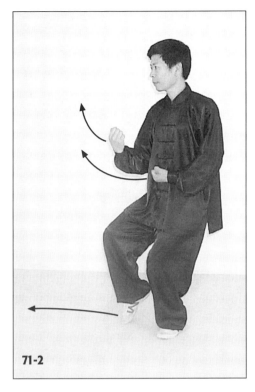

71-2

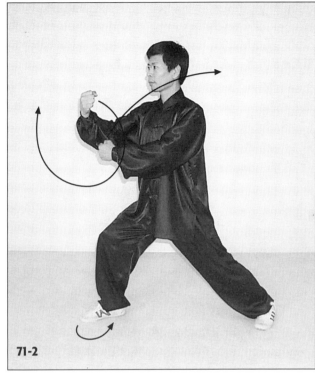

71-2

☑ Key Points

1. This is a popular Chen-style posture. You should straighten your left leg and turn your body to the right swiftly to exert the force.

2. Do not lean forward when you punch out your fists. Remember, the power is coming from your legs and waist.

3. Keep your left fist slightly behind your right fist. Push your left fist forward to assist the right-hand strike.

4. Face 8 o'clock in the final position.

☑ Self-Defense Application

Grasp your attacker's arm with both hands and pull to your lower left. Turn both hands into fists, with your right fist punching at the chest and your left punching at the belly.

Posture 72

GRASP BIRD'S TAIL–LEFT

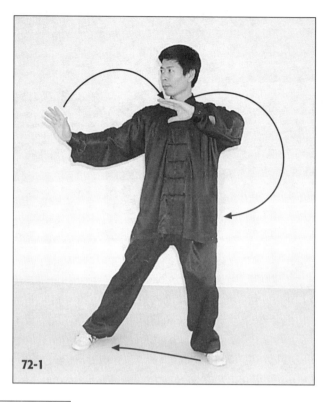

72-1

Movement 1

Shift your weight onto your left leg and turn your right toes inward, while turning your body to the left, to 6 o'clock. Open both fists and move your left hand up and to the left at shoulder level, with the palm facing down. At the same time, move your right hand to your left, then down in a counterclockwise circle to the right at the waist level, with the palm turning up.

72-2

Movement 2

Shift your weight back to your right leg and draw your left foot next to your right, toes touching the floor. Move your left hand down and to the right, to the right side of your waist, with the palm facing up, while circling your right hand up in front of your right chest with the palm facing down to form a hold-ball position. Look at your right hand.

Movement 3

Turn your body slightly to the left and step your left foot to 2 o'clock. Continue turning your body to the left to 3 o'clock and shift your weight onto your left leg to form a left bow stance. Move your left forearm up to shoulder level, with your palm facing inward and your elbow bending as if warding off a coming attack, while dropping your right hand slowly to the side of your right hip, with the palm facing down. Look at your left forearm.

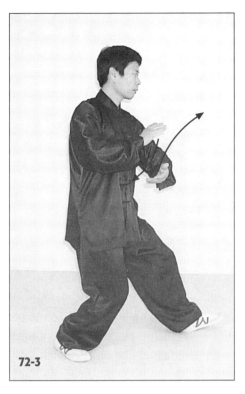

72-3

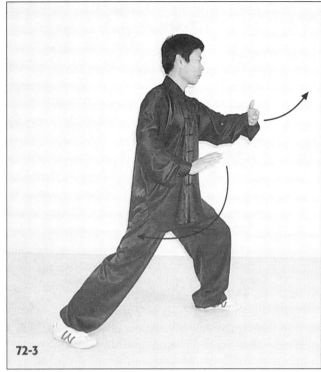

72-3

✔️ Key Points

1. Make sure your left heel touches the floor first when taking the left step. As your body weight shifts forward, press down your left sole to make your whole left foot touch the floor.

2. Keep both arms rounded. Keep your shoulders and elbows sunk.

3. Coordinate your hands' separation with your body's turning and your left leg's bending.

4. Keep a 12-inch transverse distance between your feet when forming the bow stance.

5. Face 3 o'clock in the final position.

✔️ Self-Defense Application

This is called the "Ward Off" movement. Use your left forearm to intercept your

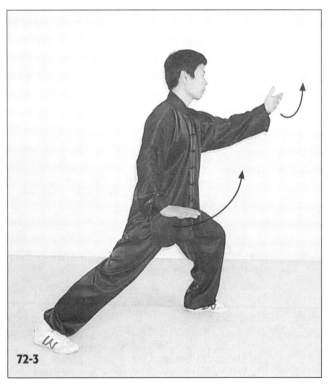

72-3

attacker's hand and dissolve the force by turning your body to the left. Bring your right arm down and pluck your hand to protect yourself from your attacker's kick.

Grasp Bird's Tail is composed of four techniques: ward off, roll back, press and push. They are linked together to deflect an attack, and to pull or push an attacker off balance.

Movement 4

Turn your body slightly to the left, to a position between 2 and 3 o'clock, and extend your left hand forward, with the palm turning down as if grabbing something. Turn your right palm up and forward, and bring your right hand up across your abdomen until it is just below your left forearm. Then, turn your body slowly to the right, to 5 o'clock, and shift your weight back to your right leg. At the same time, pull both hands back, down, up, and to the right, in a curve, until your right hand is at shoulder level with the palm facing up, and your left hand is in front of your chest with the palm facing inward. Your eyes should follow your right hand.

✔ Key Points

1. Pull back both arms in a circular movement as your body turns and your weight shifts back.

2. Keep your left foot flat on the floor. Do not lean your body forward or protrude your

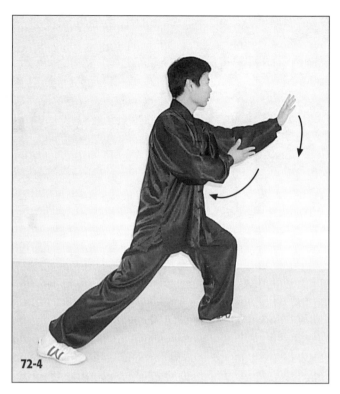

72-4

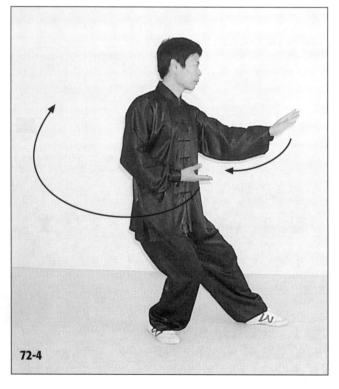

72-4

buttocks. Maintain your body in the center and root your feet into the ground to keep them solid and your body flexible.

3. Face 5 o'clock in the final position.

✔ Self-Defense Application

This is called a "Roll Back" movement. It allows you to hold your attacker's elbow and wrist to destroy balance. The pulling is energized through turning your waist and shifting your body weight backward.

Movement 5

Turn your body slowly to the left, to 3 o'clock. Bend your right arm and bring your right hand to the inside of your left wrist. Shift your body weight back to your left leg into a left bow stance while pressing both hands forward with your left palm facing inward and your right palm facing outward. Look at your left wrist.

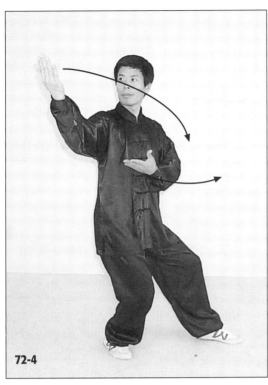

72-4

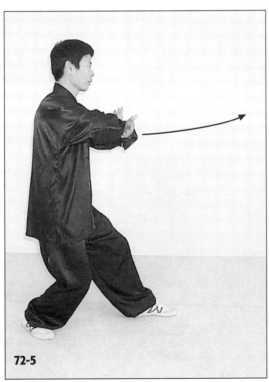

72-5

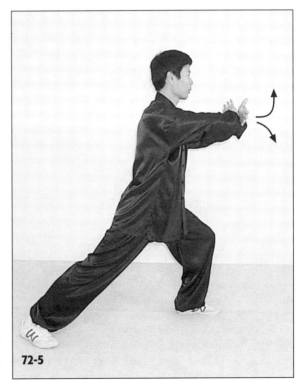

72-5

☑ Key Points

1. Pressing your hands forward must be coordinated with your body turning and your weight shifting forward. The pressing force comes from your waist and spine, in addition to your body weight. Press with a continuous pressure.

2. Keep both arms rounded and relaxed. Keep a 1-inch distance between your palms. Keep both shoulders sunk.

3. Keep your body erect. Do not lean forward when your hands press out. Keep both feet flat on the floor.

4. Face 3 o'clock in the final position.

☑ Self-Defense Application

This is called the "Press Out" movement. Use the flow of your body weight to press your left hand and forearm against your attacker's chest.

Movement 6

Following the press out motion, separate your hands to a shoulder-width and turn both palms forward and down. Sit back and shift your weight onto your right leg, raising up your left toes. At the same time, draw both hands back and down in a curve to the front of your abdomen, with the palms pressing down. Transfer your body weight slowly onto your left leg, while pushing both palms forward and upward in a curve to shoulder level. Bend your left knee to form a left bow stance. Look to the front. Arrows in bottom photograph on

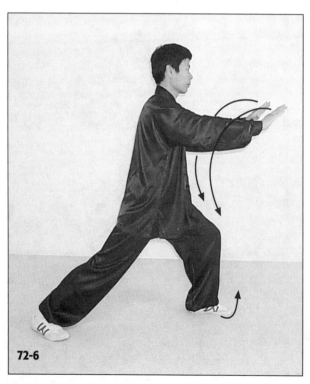

72-6

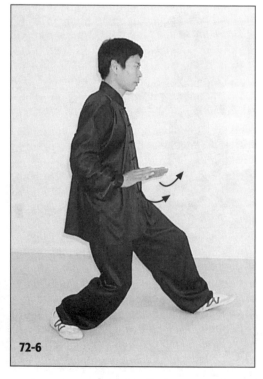

72-6

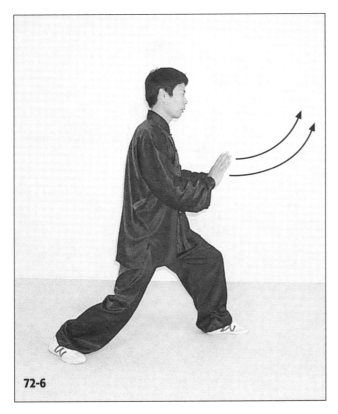

72-6

72-6

page 223 show transition to Posture 73.

✔️ Key Points

1. Keep your waist and hips relaxed. Do not shrug your shoulder when pushing out your hands. Keep your elbows slightly down.

2. Coordinate your hands pushing with your body shifting forward. Use your body to generate the push instead of your arms.

3. Do not push your body weight too far forward. Your left knee should be behind the left toes.

4. Face 3 o'clock in the final position.

✔️ Self-Defense Application

This is called the "Push Out" movement. Sit back and draw your hands back to avoid an attack. Then, pin your attacker's arms down and push toward his chest. Push upward and forward to destroy balance.

Posture 73

CROSS HANDS

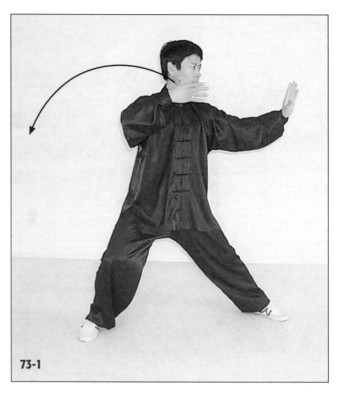

73-1

Movement 1

Rotate your right toes toward 6 o'clock, as you sit back and shift your body weight onto your right leg. Turn your body to the right, to 5 o'clock, with your left toes turning toward 6 o'clock. At the same time, move your right hand in a horizontal curve at shoulder level to your right side, with the right palm turning slowly outward and downward. Look at your right hand.

Movement 2

Shift your body weight slowly onto your left leg and bring your right foot toward your left foot, so they are parallel and a shoulder-width apart. Straighten both legs gradually and move both hands down in a vertical curve to cross at the wrist in front of your abdomen. Then move your hands up to shoulder level with your left hand nearer your body, palms facing inward. Look to the front.

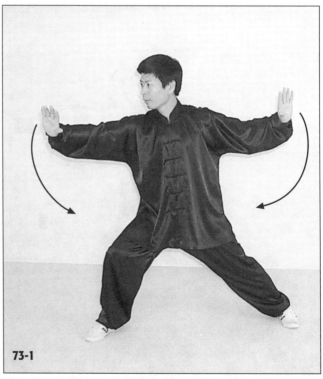

73-1

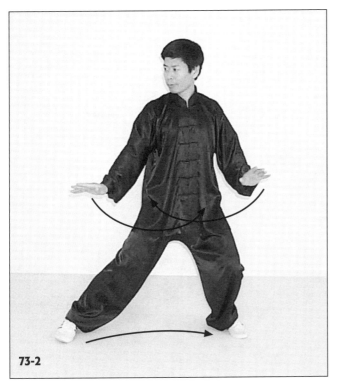

73-2

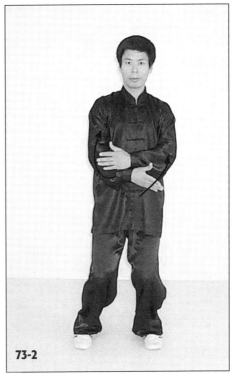

73-2

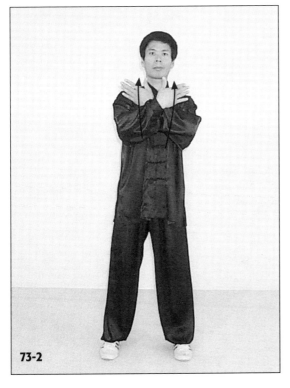

73-2

☑ Key Points

1. Place your weight evenly on both legs as your hands cross. Keep both arms in an arc shape, with elbows slightly bent.

2. Keep your body erect as you straighten your legs.

3. Face 6 o'clock in the final position.

☑ Self-Defense Application

As you sit back and turn to the right, pull and grab your left hand to deflect an attack. Bring both hands down in a circular motion and then up to protect your front body.

225

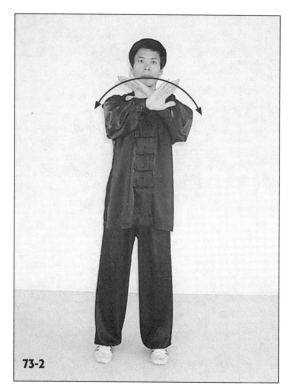

73-2

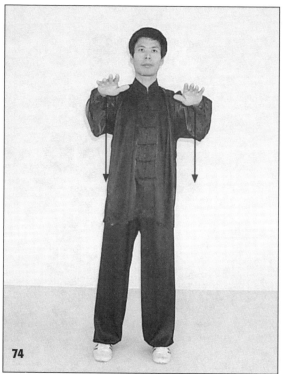

74

Posture 74

CLOSING FORM

Rotate both arms inward and turn the palms down. Separate your hands to a shoulder-width, with the fingers pointing forward. Drop both hands gradually along the side of your hips. Bring your left foot next to your right foot. Look to the front.

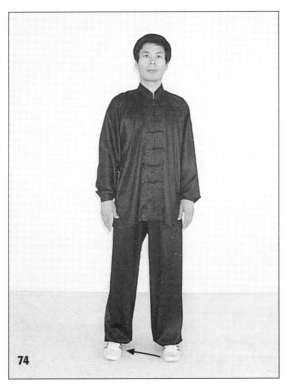

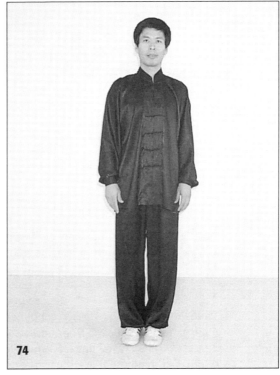

74

74

☑ Key Points

Keep your whole body relaxed. Take a deep breath and exhale slowly. Stand for a moment to feel the energy flowing in your body. Concentrate on your lower abdomen.

Postscript

We are now living in a fast-paced lifestyle. Stress becomes part of our common life events. It leads to many of our health problems, such as a headache, stiff neck, nagging backache, upset stomach, fatigue, colds, and heart disease. Stress can also make us become irritable and intolerant of even minor disturbances. Compact Tai Chi is a natural solution for stress. It uses the body's soft flow motion to soothe our mind and uses our mind meditation to relax our body. Mind plays a major role in Compact Tai Chi exercise. Our mind provides guidance for our inner energy flow. There is a new study called "psychoneuroimmunology" on how our emotions and thoughts affect our health. Our mind can trigger our body to produce a natural substance for fortifying our immune system, fighting illness, and speeding healing.

American culture is not geared toward taking an hour a day to meditate. However, if we have ten minutes, we have time to rejuvenate our body and mind through Compact Tai Chi.

Tai Chi is a life-long practice. Anyone can learn it, regardless of his or her age or athletic ability. It is convenient and cost-effective. We can practice Tai Chi anytime, anywhere. It does not require any special equipment or facility. We don't stop exercising because we are getting older; we become older because we stop exercising. I hope that readers will use Compact Tai Chi as a life-long practice to fight off the ravages of modern stress, for it leads to a longer and more fruitful life.

About the Author

*J*esse Tsao, Tai Chi master and alternative medicine and wellness consultant, specializes in the areas of relaxation, stress management, mind and body wellness, self-healing, and preventive therapies. He came to the United States in 1987, and has dedicated his life to teaching Tai Chi to promote health. He has been teaching Tai Chi for the Arizona state employee wellness program since 1994. Contracted with PJRR Health Promotion System & Consulting firm, he has been teaching Tai Chi as an alternative medicine for CIGNA HealthCare since 1997. He has also conducted Tai Chi wellness workshops, seminars, and classes for the Arizona Supreme Court, Arizona State University, the City of Phoenix Park and Recreation Department, Maricopa County Hospital, HUMANA HealthCare, Just for Women Fitness Center, Phoenix Yanxin Qigong Association, and the Scripps Center for Integrative Medicine in San Diego. He is also the founder and president of the Compact Tai Chi Healthway Club, and has lectured and demonstrated various Tai Chi forms for a local TV station. Born and trained in China, he has been practicing Wushu and Tai Chi for more than 32 years. He is currently the Director of Mind-Body Energetics at the Shi-ho Center for Creative and Healing Arts in Del Mar, California.